In memory of E. C. R.

**Longman Group Limited**
Longman House, Burnt Mill, Harlow
Essex CM20 2JE, England
Associated companies throughout the world

*Published in the United States of America
by Longman Inc., New York*

© Anthony Reading 1983

All rights reserved; no part of this publication may be
reproduced, stored in a retrieval system, or transmitted
in any form or by any means, electronic, mechanical,
photocopying, recording, or otherwise, without the
prior written permission of the Publisher.

First published 1983

**British Library Cataloguing in Publication Data**
Reading, Anthony
  Psychological aspects of pregnancy. – (Longman
  applied psychology)
  1. Pregnancy – Psychological aspects
  2. Childbirth – Psychological aspects
  I. Title
  618.2′001′9      RG560

ISBN 0-582-29614-5

**Library of Congress Cataloging in Publication Data**
Reading, Anthony.
  Psychological aspects of pregnancy.

  (Longman applied psychology)
  Bibliography: p.
  Includes index.
  1. Pregnancy – Psychological aspects.
2. Mother and child. I. Title. II. Series.
[DNLM: 1. Pregnancy. 2. Psychology. WQ 200    P973]
RG560.R4    1983        618.2′001′9      82-17146
ISBN 0-582-29614-5

Set in 10/11pt Linotron 202 Times
Printed in Hong Kong by
Astros Printing Ltd.

# Contents

| | |
|---|---|
| *Editor's preface* | vi |
| *Acknowledgements* | viii |
| 1 Introduction: pregnancy in the twentieth century | 1 |
| 2 The effects of anxiety during pregnancy | 10 |
| 3 Health beliefs and health behaviour | 25 |
| 4 The evolution of maternal feelings | 43 |
| 5 Antenatal foetal diagnosis: the woman's perspective | 53 |
| 6 The pain of labour | 70 |
| 7 Bonding: reactions to the neonate | 88 |
| 8 The postpartum and beyond | 103 |
| *References* | 111 |
| *Index* | 126 |

# Editor's preface

In most areas of applied psychology there is no shortage of hardback textbooks many hundreds of pages in length. They give a broad coverage of the total field but rarely in sufficient detail in any one topic area for undergraduates, particularly honours students. This is even more true for trainees and professionals in such areas as clinical psychology.

The Longman Applied Psychology series consists of authoritative short books each concerned with a specific aspect of applied psychology. The brief given to the authors of this series was to describe the current state of knowledge in the area, how that knowledge is applied to the solution of practical problems and what new developments of real-life relevance may be expected in the near future. The twelve books which have been commissioned so far are concerned mainly with clinical psychology, defined very broadly. Topics range from gambling to ageing and from the chemical control of behaviour to social factors in mental illness.

The books go into sufficient depth for the needs of students at all levels and professionals yet remain well within the grasp of the interested general reader. A number of groups will find their educational and professional needs or their personal interests met by this series: professional psychologists and those in training (clinical, educational, occupational, etc.); psychology undergraduates; undergraduate students in other disciplines which include aspects of applied psychology (e.g. social administration, sociology, management and particularly medicine); professionals and trainee professionals in fields outside psychology, but which draw on applications of psychology (doctors of all kinds, particularly psychiatrists and general practitioners, social workers, nurses, particularly psychiatric nurses, counsellors – such as school, vocational and marital, personnel managers).

Finally, members of the general public who have been introduced to a particular topic by the increasing number of well-informed and well-presented newspaper articles and television programmes will be able to follow it up and pursue it in more depth.

Philip Feldman

# Acknowledgements

We are indebted to the following for permission to reproduce copyright material:

The C. V. Mosby Co for a short extract from an article by Dr Weinstein 'Breast Milk – A Natural Resource' p. 973 in *American Journal of Obstetrics & Gynecology* **136**(8); Williams & Wilkins Co (Baltimore) for a short extract from an article by Mead and Newton p. 211 in *Childbearing: Its Social & Psychological Aspects* eds S. A. Richardson and A. F. Guttmacher 1967.

Chapter 1

# Introduction: pregnancy in the twentieth century

Becoming pregnant is a major transition in the female life cycle, with the prospect of assuming an additional caretaking role. It is not uncommonly associated with mixed emotions – a fulfilment of needs and desires that at the same time, may give rise to a host of conflicts and anxieties. The woman is faced with a situation which will change her life for ever: there will be changes in the family unit, changes in sex role from predominantly heterosexual to maternal, and possibly a substantial loss of freedom. Reactions to the pregnancy will be shaped by a multitude of factors. The woman's past and present circumstances, her desire to take on the role of motherhood, the level of support available and her attitude towards the pregnancy. Her partner's attitude will be also important, where she is relying upon him for support/parenting. It is clear that for a proportion of women, pregnancy and all this entails constitutes a major life stress. Surveys have found that women with children and with few social supports or economic resources have an increased incidence of depression, leading the authors to conclude that childbearing is one of the risk factors for depression (Brown and Harris 1978).

# 2  Psychological aspects of pregnancy

## Taking control

With the accessibility of effective, if not ideal, contraceptives, increasing control is being exercised over the reproductive process. It is now necessary for the woman using contraceptives to take an initial decision to become pregnant, to have her intrauterine contraceptive device (IUCD) removed, to discard her diaphragm or discontinue the pill. This will be straightforward in the case of self-administered methods, although it will not be obvious to the man. Discontinuing the condom is a more visible decision, while the IUCD requires forward planning, since a visit to a health professional is required. Although we now enjoy the capacity to control our fertility, evidence suggests this may not be exercised in quite the rational way this knowledge permits. For example, Cartwright (1976) found 6 per cent of married primiparae were pleased on discovering they were pregnant, 10 per cent would have preferred it to have happened earlier, 19 per cent felt it had happened too soon and did not want to become pregnant, and 4 per cent were sorry it had happened at all. Taking both multiparae and primiparae together, only 52 per cent described the pregnancy as intended, non accidental and were pleased it had happened.

A further group for whom pregnancy may not be a uniformly positive realization is the young. The problem of teenage pregnancy in both the United Kingdom and the United States is a growing concern in view of the medical risks and psychological and social sequelae. The failure of this group to obtain adequate contraceptive cover is likely to be the product of many factors. The belief 'it won't happen to me'; the concern that obtaining contraception will have connotations of promiscuity, 'nice girls don't'; the fear parents will find out; the alienation felt toward the family planning clinics, which may be staffed by predominantly middle-aged, middle-class women, perceived to have little in common; the fear of having to undergo pelvic examination and a host of other factors may contribute to prevent contraception being obtained. Having become pregnant, a proportion go on to receive a termination of pregnancy. For some this is not an available option, either for religious or moral reasons, or because they wait too long before seeking medical help. Denial of pregnancy is not common but is seen, even to the extent of arriving at the casualty department with acute stomach cramps which on examination are discovered to be contractions!

## Fertility patterns

The control of fertility permits a woman to postpone childbearing until she believes herself ready to embark upon this life change. Such increased fertility control has implications for women who fail to become pregnant on suspending contraceptive use. It is a tragic irony for a woman to discover her infertility after a decade of diligent contraceptive use. Women are most receptive to impregnation in their late teens and early twenties. The likelihood of becoming pregnant each cycle, assuming sexual activity, declines during the second and third decades. While a woman may become pregnant almost immediately at 20, it may require many more cycles beyond the age of 30.

Information on innate human fertility comes from studies on fecundability – or the probability of conception per menstrual cycle. Vincent (1961) studied the fecundability of 15,000 women who were contestants in a family competition in France after the First World War. He found this to rise from 15 per cent at 16 to 24 per cent at the age of 18–19 and to increase more slowly to 27 per cent at age 25. Since this information is derived from surveys of newlyweds, these should be regarded as maximal values, assuming a highest frequency of intercourse. MacLeod and Gold (1953) studied 428 New York women who were trying to conceive and found that, while 83 per cent were pregnant within six months at intercourse frequencies of 4 or more per week, the rate dropped progressively to 51 per cent at frequencies of 3–4 per week and 32 per cent at 1–2 times per week.

In addition to the natural decline in reproductive functioning, delaying childbearing may lead to additional problems. A number of diseases may reduce fertility and postponing childbearing increases the likelihood, statistically at least, of these being contracted. Pelvic inflammatory disease (PID) is of concern, since it can lead to occlusion of the Fallopian tubes and infertility. The greater incidence of veneral disease has increased these problems, as have certain contraceptive methods. Infertility secondary to a termination of pregnancy has been documented, and IUCDs have been associated with an increased likelihood of PID, since it is believed that the thread attached to the IUCD may provide a vehicle for bacteria to pass from the vagina to the uterus, thereby facilitating the spread of infection.

## The failure to conceive

These factors combined indicate the concern over the act of conception and demonstrate that this should not be regarded as an inevitability. One in ten couples will have to confront the realization of infertility and in spite of recent advances in treatment, in the form of artificial insemination by donor (AID), test-tube babies (*in vitro* fertilization) tubal reconstruction by microsurgery and fertility drugs, for some the solution will be elusive. Psychological causes of infertility have been examined. Evidence has been drawn from the occurrence of the so-called 'ramp' pregnancy, referring to the woman who becomes pregnant after attending an infertility clinic and before the instigation of active treatment. Similarly, it has been claimed that infertile women may become pregnant following an adoption. The argument has been that the relief of tension and anxiety occasioned by the clinic visit or the adopted baby leads to a spontaneous pregnancy. However, on scrutiny this data is suspect. Bias is introduced by memory factors and, in the case of the ramp pregnancy, the likelihood that the visit to the specialist coincides with a period of peak motivation, so that other factors may be optimum at this time. For example, the couple may be engaging in intercourse more frequently. That the psyche is able to exert a profound influence on reproductive functioning is not in dispute, since the female reproductive system circuitry is vulnerable to its effects at every point. In extreme cases, psychological stress may produce amenorrhoea or anovulatory cycles. Difficulties arise with the attempt to identify the specific effects of precise psychological states, since methodological problems confound much of the data in this area.

Whatever the aetiological role, once a problem has been recognized, psychological factors may assume importance. The conscious act of stopping a contraceptive method may inhibit sexual feelings or arouse anxiety as pregnancy is awaited. A fear of failure may then develop. Infertility investigations may themselves cause problems, because these tend to be intrusive. Sexual activity may be put on a schedule, permitted after an abstinence period and in accordance with the woman's temperature chart. Sexual problems may develop owing to the strain of complying with these instructions. We have seen male impotence result from having to keep a daily record of sexual behaviour and so the potentially disruptive effects of such investigations should be appreciated. It is necessary for infertility clinics to attend to the psychological aspects of both the treatment and the investigations they provide.

## Elective childlessness

In considering psychological aspects of pregnancy, it is important to acknowledge that not all couples want or intend to have children. While such attitudes may change over time, surveys have consistently identified a proportion for whom childlessness is a rational option. It is necessary to distinguish between intentional childlessness and postponement of childbearing until a more optimum time. Unfortunately, the latter may lead to unintentional childlessness, owing to the increased difficulties in achieving reproduction later in life. This leads to a consideration of the motives for childbearing. There are many candidates, although the evidence for innate drives is weak. The considerable social and cultural pressure to become parents needs to be acknowledged since many Western societies may be characterized as 'child centred'. Greene (1963), writing an article entitled 'I don't want to be a mother,' remarked that 'stating such a preference was met with as much shock as if she had announced she was running for the Communist party cell block in her basement!' Many couples in developing and developed countries become parents for economic reasons and as a means of safe-guarding themselves in their old age. The evidence that having children makes the marriage happier is inconclusive, with the data tending to favour increased stability but not necessarily happiness.

## The changing face of obstetrics

Having become pregnant, a woman is now confronted with the fruits of high-technology antenatal and obstetric care. This area has changed dramatically during the last twenty years and while increased reliance on technology and active intervention has been accompanied by reductions in perinatal mortality rates, concern has been expressed over the social and psychological implications of the way in which childbirth is currently being managed. Simply pointing to the fall in perinatal mortality is in itself insufficient justification, since many other factors have contributed to these changes. Even if obstetric practice had continued unaltered, these rates would have continued to fall because of the relatively greater decline in fertility rates among those at greatest risk of maternal and perinatal death. Improved health and socio-economic conditions have also had widespread beneficial effects.

Critics argue that there exists a law of diminishing returns, with the complications of prophylaxis ultimately outstripping or becoming worse than the original problem. For example, Neutra *et al.* (1978) have estimated that the absolute benefit of electronic foetal monitoring in labour on neonatal death rates was of the order of one life saved for every 1,000 babies monitored. Such gains must be offset against the social and psychological burden imposed on the woman by such devices. While such changes in obstetric practice may be viewed positively, since the motives are undoubtedly sound, concern has been expressed at the degree to which the pendulum may have swung too far, so that the routine use of technological intervention has had the effect of dehumanizing and depersonalizing the woman's experience of delivery (Turnbull 1977).

## An ethnographic perspective

Pregnancy and childbirth have evolved from being predominantly natural functions to ones controlled by the medical profession and defined accordingly, within this frame of reference, as medical problems. As Oakley (1977) has commented, 'childbirth has changed from being managed by lay women to being controlled by professionally trained men!' Such changes have been reflected also in the location of birth, since the trend towards hospital delivery has increased. In 1927 hospital confinements constituted about 15 per cent of all live births, in 1946, 54 per cent and in 1972, 91 per cent. In the USA by 1944, 74 per cent of babies were delivered in hospitals. Management of childbirth has changed accordingly, with the pregnant woman now treated as if she were sick, and rules governing the management of hospital patients applied to her. Such a perspective sanctions a passive role for the woman, attended by 'experts', who will take whatever action is necessary. Oakley (1977) has contrasted Western obstetric practices with those occurring in preliterate societies. She observes that, in addition to where the birth occurs and who controls it, the position adopted by the woman at birth has changed from predominantly vertical (in 62 out of 76 non-European societies) to the supine in hospital deliveries. This preference for a reclining position has been considered by Mead and Newton (1967) as a consequence of casting the pregnant woman in a sick role, so that the delivery is viewed as a surgical procedure: 'The position of the woman at birth is arranged as nearly as possible to conform to this concept. Her body is flat and her neck is straight without a pillow to support it, as is the custom on operating tables. Her legs are mechanically spread wide apart with leg braces to allow the physician to have an unobstructed view of the perineum' (p. 211). Although these comments are not valid today in their entity, since stirrups are rarely used in the UK, other than for stitching and instrumental deliveries, they do serve to illustrate the passive role assigned to the woman, and the way in which the delivery has been shaped by normative medical practice.

## Towards a behavioural perspective of pregnancy and childbirth

The process of pregnancy contains many more features of psychological interest than can possibly be included in a book of this size. Increasing attention is being given to behavioural aspects of pregnancy in influencing obstetric outcome. This will be reflected in the following pages, since the topics to be dealt with are those considered amenable to both empirical study and psychological intervention. This is in accordance with a more widespread recognition of the importance of the effect of life-style factors on physical morbidity. As Stachnik (1980) has forcefully stated: 'The health of Americans is a function of our behaviour, what we choose to eat and drink, and the nature of our environment.' In which case, physical problems may be regarded as, within certain physiological limits, behavioural problems requiring the alteration of characteristic response patterns. Thus, anxiety, health behaviour and beliefs and pain in childbirth are all important in determining obstetric outcome, and may also be considered from a behavioural standpoint, whereby behavioural intervention may improve perinatal morbidity. Such a perspective recognizes the limitations of viewing psychological processes divorced from physiology, and so attention will be given to physiological issues where this is felt to be appropriate. The chapters are organized around discrete problem areas, with their selection reflecting the author's current interests.

Chapter 2

# The effects of anxiety during pregnancy

## Introduction

There has been considerable research relating the psychological state of the woman during pregnancy to the delivery experience and the likelihood of obstetric complications. As Ferreira (1969) has remarked, 'The belief that the emotional attitudes and behavior of the pregnant woman may affect the child she carries is apparently as old as the human race.' From the Bible onwards, it has been accepted that a woman's psychological experience during pregnancy will directly affect the functioning and anatomy of her unborn child. For example, birthmarks have been attributed to maternal impressions (emotional or visual stimuli) experienced during the pregnancy (Ferreira 1969). Although the adverse effects of anxiety on the pregnant woman may have been recognized for many years (Ferreira 1965), attempts to document this influence are more recent. Anxiety has been studied in relation to foetal growth retardation, antenatal complications, premature onset of labour, intrapartum and postpartum complications and subsequent mother-neonate interaction. This evidence will be examined in this chapter in order to elaborate a framework to understand the way in which anxiety may have an effect. A concluding section will consider clinical implications, since if anxiety can be shown to be an important factor, it follows that psychological methods of anxiety management may be relevant to antenatal care.

## The effects of anxiety: research strategies

A number of research strategies have been utilized in studying the effects of anxiety on pregnancy. These can be ranked by degree of scientific rigour and are: (1) anecdotal case material; (2) the study of the incidence of complications in women who have had stressful psychiatric disorders; (3) the assessment of women experiencing particular complications in an attempt to identify predisposing characteristics; (4) an extension of the third strategy which has consisted of a comparison of the response profiles of different patient groups defined by complication; (5) the study of multiple complications whereby complications have been viewed as the result of a unitary process, and the response profiles of women with complications compared with those undergoing uncomplicated pregnancies and deliveries.

The limitations of drawing inferences and conclusions from unsubstantiated clinical case material are well recognized and will not be discussed at length here. Similarly, problems exist with research on women with previous psychiatric histories. Research has shown that such women produce a disproportionate number of low birthweight infants. However, they may also differ in other ways, in addition to their stress or anxiety levels, since patients who have had a stressful psychiatric disorder will constitute a heterogeneous sample, with considerable variation in terms of nutritional status, the use of psychotropic medication and their adherence to antenatal health care recommendations. Moreover, this research begs the question as to the nature of the stress, since this remains unspecified. The third strategy, research assessing the effects of anxiety on single complications, has generally yielded unimpressive results. Sample sizes have typically been small, the measures used often psychometrically wanting, as with projective testing, and the premise (that a group defined by the presence of a single complication, such as hyperemesis gravidarum, habitual abortion, toxaemia, prematurity or labour difficulties, may be treated as a homogeneous entity) an untested assumption. Attention will be confined here to multiple complication studies as these have generally yielded the most impressive results.

## The evidence

A series of related studies by McDonald (1968) has documented the presence of increased anxiety in complicated pregnancies. For example, a positive correlation between duration of labour and anxiety was reported in a survey of eighty-six Caucasian married women of mixed parity. Anxiety scores on the Manifest Anxiety Scale (MAS) were also found to be higher in women experiencing abnormal deliveries (McDonald and Christakos 1963; McDonald and Parham 1964). Unfortunately, the interpretation of these findings is complicated by the late stage in pregnancy at which anxiety was assessed and because, in at least one study, antenatal anxiety was assessed retrospectively following the birth. A further difficulty derives from the degree to which scores on the MAS reflect enduring personality traits rather than elevations in state anxiety occurring in response to the events of pregnancy. The importance of drawing a distinction between trait and state components of anxiety will be returned to later in this chapter.

Gorsuch and Key (1974) administered the state anxiety scale of the State Trait Anxiety Inventory (Spielberger *et al.* 1970) to a group of 118 women serially over the course of the pregnancy. Women with abnormal pregnancies showed increased state anxiety during the third and fourth months. Stressful life events were also measured, with an association between problem pregnancies and increased life event scores during the six months prior to delivery. Delivery complications were associated with higher anxiety scores on a standardized measure of personality (IPAT), measured during the third trimester in a survey of 146 women (Crandon 1979). Of this sample, 34 were identified as displaying high anxiety, with a greater proportion of complications occurring in this group. It is regrettable that no information was provided on other characteristics of this sample which could have selectively influenced outcome. Once again, the late stage in pregnancy at which the anxiety assessments were conducted raises the possibility that the women may have become anxious through becoming aware of the problematic status of their pregnancy, in which case the pre-existing obstetric problem may have been instrumental in influencing outcome.

Inconsistent results have also emerged. Thus Burstein *et al.* (1974) administered the MAS to 61 women between 36 and 38 weeks gestation. Of their sample, 24 labours were described as complicated with no differences emerging between the groups of women experiencing complicated or uncomplicated labours with respect to antenatal anxiety scores. Edwards and Jones (1970) reported a differential pattern in state anxiety on the STAI according to whether a normal or complicated delivery had occurred. Of the 53 women having normal deliveries, state anxiety remained low until near delivery (within two weeks), at which time anxiety levels rose. The converse pattern emerged for those women experiencing complications, as anxiety remained at a lower level until near the time of delivery, when their anxiety decreased. Finally, Beck *et al.* (1980) administered the state anxiety scale on two occasions – during the third trimester of pregnancy and at the time of admission to the labour room. None of the measures collected prior to the delivery predicted the likelihood of complications as a whole, although state anxiety on admission was predictive of length of labour.

Research concerned with the effects of stressful life events on pregnancy outcome is also relevant, in so far as such events may lead to elevations in state anxiety. For example, Nuckolls *et al.* (1972) measured adaptive potential for pregnancy by asking about the following categories: self- and ego-strength, marriage, the support of the extended family, social resources and the nature of the pregnancy in terms of whether it was planned, and feelings towards forthcoming events. Women completed an inventory of recent stressful life events in the thirty-second week of pregnancy and these scores were related to complication rates. Out of the 360 women initially studied, complete data were available for 237. No significant associations between stressful life event scores and complication rates were found. However, examining subdivisions, in terms of mounting life change before and during pregnancy, the women with both high stress scores and social assets were found to have a reduced incidence of complications. This suggests that the adverse effects of stress during pregnancy may be offset by the adequacy of the social support system available. Discrepant results were obtained by Jones (1979), since low scores on a life event inventory were associated with higher complication rates. The author of this study speculated that exposure to life stress had an innoculating effect, which prepared the woman for the delivery experience. Such a model, whereby moderate levels of anxiety facilitate adjustment, has been proposed in the context of pre-operative anxiety (Janis 1958), although Jones's (1979) failure to study other factors, such as level of psychosocial support available, limits the generalizations which may be drawn. Moreover, this finding may reflect the special circumstances of the delivery for the women studied, since they were admitted two weeks prior to the date of delivery – a practice acknowledged to be highly stressful for the patients, 'many of whom were young and away from home for the first time, often leaving a spouse and sometimes other children at home' (p. 408). Such conditions cannot be considered representative of customary obstetric practice, casting doubt on the relevance of the study's findings.

Life events have been studied in relation to prematurity. Williams *et al.* (1975) studied 46 women, 22 per cent of whom delivered prematurely. Following the delivery, women were asked to report on life events during the pregnancy. A comparable increase in life events was reported by both term and pre-term groups, although stress scores were elevated in both groups compared to pre-conception. Retrospective assessments were also used by Newton *et al.* (1979) in a survey at 132 women, who were required to report the occurrence of life events within each trimester. Three study groups were defined by weeks of gestation: 83 at full term, 30 pre-term and 19 very pre-term. Higher numbers of life events were reported by pre-term women in the week preceding labour.

## Methodological considerations

Before considering the mechanisms of the effect of anxiety on perinatal outcome, a number of methodological issues will be raised. Rather than address problems related to individual studies, a number of general points will be made in order to guide future research. There are four main issues:

1. *Specification of the sample*: essential information on the sample characteristics, in terms of socio-demographic details as well as previous and current obstetric history, is often omitted. It is necessary to

provide such data and to establish, whenever possible, obstetrically homogeneous samples, since this will facilitate data interpretation. An adequate sample size will assist in determining the contribution of anxiety *vis à vis* the many other influences on outcome.
2. *Predictive measures*: the variation in measures utilized, as well as the stage at which these are administered, limits the generalizations which can be drawn. A fundamental problem has been the failure to make explicit the aspect of anxiety under investigation. The distinction between transitory state anxiety and individual differences in anxiety proneness, or trait anxiety, is an important one, since they may have differential impact on different stages of pregnancy.
3. *Selection of dependent measures*: related to (2) is the need to study the effects of anxiety on aspects of care which are representative and have clinical significance. It should be acknowledged that many of these will be inter-related, with insufficient knowledge about factors influencing these processes.
4. *Repeated measures designs*: in order to obtain an adequate evaluation of state anxiety it is necessary to measure this repeatedly throughout the pregnancy. Measures obtained late in pregnancy may be influenced by psychological and bodily changes that have taken place. Thus, anxiety may be engendered by the woman perceiving the concern displayed by the obstetrician.

## Explanatory mechanisms

If anxiety has an effect, through what mechanism is this exerted? Similarly, not all complications are equally vulnerable to the effects of anxiety and so it is necessary to identify those which are particularly sensitive. Experimental studies on animals have documented the deleterious effects of stressful environments on neuroendocrine processes in the mother and foetus, both during pregnancy and on subsequent development. Research on humans has to date yielded equivocal findings, although many of the studies must be considered inadequate, owing to the serious methodological problems.

## The benefits of anxiety

Anxiety has not always been thought of as increasing risk. Early research tended to view anxiety as adaptive in preparing the woman for delivery and motherhood. This followed from the view of pregnancy as a developmental stage, placing great demands on the coping resources of the woman (Bibring 1959; Breen 1975), with the ensuing adaptational process, through the elicitation of anxiety, preparing for motherhood. As a result, denial of the pregnancy and related conflicts were regarded as a common way of avoiding anxiety, resulting in inadequate psychological preparation (Uddenberg *et al.* 1976; Schereshefsky and Yarrow 1973). A comparable framework has been proposed to explain the benefits of a certain level of anxiety on the outcome of surgery, with Janis (1958) suggesting the existence of an optimum level of pre-operative anxiety which facilitates recovery. However, attempts to confirm this have been unsuccessful, with subsequent research concluding that the lower the pre-operative anxiety level the more favourable the response (Sime 1976; Reading 1979). As a result, a linear relationship between anxiety and complications in pregnancy will be proposed here, since this has received most consistent support from the evidence.

## Towards a conceptual framework

The model shown in Fig. 1 is an attempt to synthesize

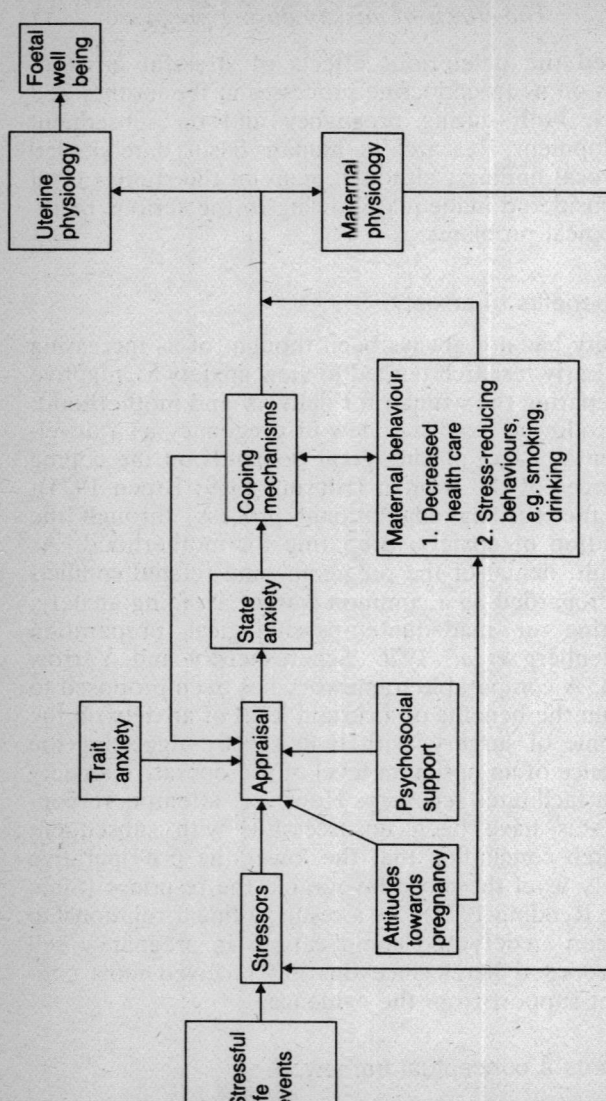

Fig. 1  The influence of maternal anxiety on the course and outcome of the pregnancy

what is known about the effects of anxiety on the course and outcome of pregnancy, thereby helping to identify clinical implications and future research objectives. Anxiety refers to state anxiety as distinct from enduring personality predispositions or traits. The model acknowledges that the impact of 'stressors', in whatever form, will be moderated by a number of factors. These will include:
(a) trait anxiety, which refers to the predisposition to react emotionally in stressful circumstances and to perceive events as threatening;
(b) attitudes held in relation to the pregnancy, since it cannot be assumed that these will be uniformly positive and, where negative or ambivalent attitudes are held, may amplify the impact of stressful life events;
(c) it is well establish that individuals differ widely in the degree to which objective circumstances are appraised as threatening. It is necessary, therefore, to allow for the woman's appraisal process in determining the impact of a 'stressor', since this will reflect the outcome of both the stress and her appreciation of the coping resources available to her to offset the difficulties encountered;
(d) related to (c) is the level of psychosocial support available to the woman. Where a woman has access to an extended social support network, this will have a protective effect;
(e) just as there are individual differences in the degree to which events are perceived as threatening, so there will be differences in the coping resources available and the effectiveness of such coping strategies, once implemented, in reducing stress.

## The effects of anxiety

It is evident that the effects of stress will be modulated

by a variety of processes. Assuming a failure in coping resources, so that a pregnant woman is exposed to prolonged stress, what will be the effects of this on uterine physiology, and by implication foetal health and development? Maternal stress will be associated with the release of catecholamines and changes in the circulating levels of adrenocorticoid steroids and other hormones. Whereas maternally-released stress hormones cross the placenta in only very limited concentrations, of the order of less than 20 per cent of their original concentration (Artal 1980), elevated levels of catecholamines in maternal circulation may exert an indirect effect. Increased anxiety may lead to increased maternal blood pressure and by implication decreased uterine blood flow, with the attendant risks of consequent foetal asphyxia (Ascher 1978) and foetal catecholamine elaboration (Fox 1979). The effects of stress on blood flow have been vividly shown by studies on rhesus monkeys. Subjecting pregnant monkeys to 'mild' stressors has resulted in a marked decrease in arterial oxygenation of the foetus (Morishima *et al.* 1978).

What if anxiety is high during or prior to labour? The adverse effects of anxiety on progress in labour have been long recognized. For example, higher plasma cortisol levels, attributable to psychological stress, have been associated with a longer duration of first-stage labour (Burns 1976). Similarly, Lederman *et al.* (1978) found elevations in maternal plasma epinephrine to be associated with lower uterine activity and with a longer duration of second-stage labour. The role of epinephrine and norepinephrine have been examined by Pancheri *et al.* (1979) by obtaining serial measures of pain, anxiety and plasma catecholamines in women defined as undergoing fast or slow labours. They found that the fast group showed higher initial levels of state anxiety and the slow group a rapid increment in anxiety levels. Labour was associated with an increment in norepinephrine levels (with corresponding increase in uterine contractility) and a lower increment in epinephrine values (with a less antagonistic effect on uterine contractility). The authors suggested that anxiety may have the function of being a neuroendocrine starter at the catecholamine level, inducing an increase in norepinephrine and maintaining it afterwards, thereby offering a rationale for the involvement of emotional arousal in the premature onset of labour, as claimed in the study by Newton *et al.* (1979). It also suggests that epinephrine, which is highly responsive to anxiety, may be an important intervening variable in impairing progress in labour. It is evident, therefore, that the release of hormones and certain biochemical processes accompanying stress are implicated in uterine functioning, and so are likely to influence the course of labour, or may have synergistic interactions with medication administered at the time. This may result in a prolongation of labour, with implications for pain levels and complications.

It is also necessary to consider the possible synergistic effects of maternal stress levels and foetal physiology. The magnitude and clinical significance of the former may be moderated by the physiological resilience of the latter. For example, the exposure of a normal pregnant woman to psychological stress has been shown to result in foetal tachycardia, persisting for about ten minutes following the cessation of the stressor (Copher and Huber 1967). Such changes in foetal cardiodynamics induced by maternal psychic stress may be on the whole transient. However, in already compromised foetuses these may have a critical bearing on outcome.

### Behavioural implications of anxiety

Figure 1 also points to the way in which anxiety may

affect foetal wellbeing indirectly through its effect on behaviour. This possibility has largely been neglected by researchers. Although the effects of behaviour during pregnancy will be dealt with in the following chapter, it should be acknowledged that stress may stimulate certain behaviour, such as smoking more heavily or turning to the solace of alcohol, which will be counter-therapeutic. Furthermore, anxiety may reduce the likelihood of compliance with health advice in terms of decreased attendance for antenatal care or birth preparation classes, through preoccupation with the source of the stress. Other effects may be in the form of accident proneness or improper diet. In extreme circumstances, anxiety may also prompt more direct action in the form of attempts to induce an abortion through the ingestion of abortifacients – the so-called 'gin binge'.

## Conclusions and implications

The associations depicted in this framework are not unidirectional, since various possible relationships between anxiety and obstetric complications exist: namely, anxiety may lead to complications, the precursor of the complication may cause the anxiety or the two may be the result of a third factor. For example, in the high-risk mother it may be difficult to distinguish between the two possible components of foetal catecholamine response – that resulting from adverse foetal circumstance arising from the medical problem and that resulting from the maternal anxiety engendered by the medical condition and its treatment (Fox 1979). Irrespective of the nature of these associations, where anxiety is raised, psychologists may have a role to play at the intervention level in the antenatal setting in order to facilitate the course of pregnancy.

For example, psychological methods of anxiety management are well established in the psychiatric setting (Rachman 1974) and their efficacy has been reported with antenatal patients (Bloom and Cantrill 1978; Kondas and Scetnicka 1972). Stress management may become a routine facility offered by antenatal clinics in which case it would be necessary to identify women displaying elevated levels of anxiety or stress at the time of their clinic visits. This could be accomplished by screening the entire population for anxiety or stressful life events (Spielberger and Jacobs 1979). This would require psychological measures which would be sufficiently sensitive and reliable to be acceptable to patients in this context. Alternatively, a number of social and demographic factors have been shown to confer increased risk of poor outcome (Feldstein and Butler 1965; Donahue and Wan 1973). It is widely appreciated that patients at the extremes of reproductive age, non-white, and of low socio-economic status are also at increased risk of poor outcome, although the determinants of poor outcome in this heterogeneous group have not yet been determined. However, whichever socio-demographic criteria are employed, so-designated high risk patients account for only half of the perinatal morbidity and mortality (Wilson and Schifrin 1980).

There is a need for large-scale prospective evaluations, monitoring anxiety and concomitant obstetric and psychological factors over the course of the pregnancy. This would determine the pattern of change and whether anxiety peaks occur for certain subgroups at different gestational stages. For example, Kumar and Robson (1978) identified a subgroup of primiparae displaying high anxiety early in the pregnancy which was found to be related to previous elective termination of pregnancy. Kumar and Robson (1978) suggested that the anxiety reflected concern over the viability of the current pregnancy in the form of a fear of retribution. In the context of a prospective study,

## 24  Psychological aspects of pregnancy

anxiety profiles could be examined in relation to the incidence of complications and outcome variables, taking into account the various medical and obstetric factors related to outcome. Such a study could be combined with a controlled evaluation of the clinical impact of a stress management programme compared to traditional bith preparation classes.

Chapter 3

# Health beliefs and health behaviour

## Introduction

The focus in this chapter will be on the behavioural aspects of pregnancy. Having become pregnant, a woman may be inundated with health advice concerning what she should and should not do. Pregnant women are advised to make a number of changes in their life style in order to ensure the optimum intra-uterine environment for the foetus. While parts of this advice have their origins in folklore and superstition, as will be seen in this chapter, much is founded on sound medical knowledge as to the hazardous effects on the foetus of certain behaviour during pregnancy.

Pregnancy necessitates intensified and protracted contact with medical agencies. During their visits women are provided with a variety of information and instruction concerning diet, smoking, alcohol consumption, medication adherence, regular clinic attendance, participation in birth preparation classes and observance of dental care, along with a range of practical preparations for the baby. In common with findings on the efficacy of health advice in other branches of medical practice, the degree to which pregnant women adhere to health advice varies considerably and is frequently less than ideal, with a proportion continuing to smoke and consume alcohol in spite of advice to the contrary (Dalby 1978).

Increasing attention is being paid to the effects of maternal behaviour, in terms of failure to comply with health advice, on the course and outcome of the pregnancy and the subsequent wellbeing of the neonate. The issues of foetal health and the viability of the pregnancy may be considered behavioural problems in instances where smoking and alcohol consumption is high, in so far as behavioural change is required on the woman's part in order to facilitate the course of pregnancy. The thesis is that while the ultimate effects of low adherence to health care advice may have physiological implications, the origin of the problem may be considered from a psychological standpoint. Such an orientation is illustrated by the title of a recent journal article, in which foetal alcohol syndrome was referred to as 'behavioral teratology' (Abel 1980).

It would be misleading to imply that health behaviours are only of interest in terms of their bearing on the pregnancy. The woman's own health will be also affected. Similarly, changes that occur during pregnancy may have benefits in the longer term, since if a woman stops smoking while she is pregnant she may not resume doing so following the delivery. This possibility will be returned to later in this chapter. For present purposes, attention will be focused on the effects of the woman's behaviour on perinatal morbidity and mortality. The behaviours to be considered are: clinic attendance, smoking, alcohol consumption, nutrition and drug use. Each of these will be considered in isolation although, as will be evident from concluding sections of the chapter, women failing to comply with one are also likely to be noncompliant in other respects. This has implications for research documenting the effects of non-compliance on the foetus: it is appropriate to consider these in combination, since smokers are also likely to be drinkers and vice versa. Having reviewed this evidence, a final section will discuss what can be done to modify behaviour and promote compliance with health advice, thereby reducing the exposure of the foetus to risk factors.

## Clinic attendance

Pregnancy necessitates early and repeated attendance of antenatal clinics. An important indication of the degree to which a woman is likely to comply with health advice may be the time at which she first attends for antenatal care. Although the benefits of early attendance are established, a substantial proportion of women fail to attend until their pregnancy is well advanced. It is ironic that such woman are very often those most likely to benefit from health advice, dietary supplements and foetal diagnosis. For example, a survey of antenatal clinic attendance in Aberdeen revealed an inverse association between social class and week of first clinic visit (MacKinlay 1970). Attendance before the seventeenth week of gestation was positively correlated with socio-economic status. There was also a tendency for young women undergoing their first pregnancy to attend after the seventeenth week.

Interestingly, a study conducted in the USA exposed an unexpected cause of late initial attendance. Quick *et al.* (1981) compared over 4,000 birth records in a Health Maintenance Organization (HMO) with 19,000 births in community settings (attending private obstetricians). There was a surprising tendency for the latter to attend earlier for antenatal care and to have fewer visits overall. This appeared to result from the HMO's administrative policy of offering appointments at a later stage of pregnancy. Such a policy may limit access to foetal screening techniques. For the population as a whole, low birthweight increased as the level of antenatal care received decreased. This finding emerged after controlling for the relevant socio-demographic and risk factors.

The stage at which booking-in takes place may be indicative of ambivalent attitudes towards the pregnancy or may simply reflect practical difficulties in attending the clinic. The former may characterize the teenage group, while the problem of disposing of the remainder of the family may constitute a deterrent for multiparae. Whatever the reason, late attendance has a number of profound implications. As will be discussed in Chapter 5, it may make the woman ineligible for antenatal diagnosis and it is the older woman for whom such procedures may have greatest relevance. Late attendance may mean that treatment of reversible problems will be delayed so that damage to the foetus results. Women may also be inadequately informed as to the need to control their drug intake and refrain from smoking and drinking.

Studies of women making appropriate use of antenatal services have shown them to be more likely to be married, have more schooling, and believe in preventive services for young children. Similarly, mothers with less than eight years of education, with similarly educated husbands, and who were less than 20 years of age, have been found to be 7.5 times more likely to receive inadequate antenatal care (Gortmaker 1979). However, it is necessary for researchers in this area to expand their focus in order to include the shortcomings of the clinics, as perceived by the woman. For many, repeated hospital attendance will be an onerous prospect, particularly as antenatal clinics, in Britain at least, may be characterized by long delays and a lack of continuity of staff contact. Providing community clinics with nursery facilities has been suggested as a possible remedy to some of these problems (Reid and McIlwaine 1980).

In addition to the procedural aspects of clinic

attendance, some women may find the content of the interviews and examinations off-putting. A proportion may experience difficulty or anxiety associated with the repeated vaginal examinations. In extreme circumstances this dislike may assume phobic proportions, although such instances may be the result of poorly managed examinations in the past (Fordney-Settlage 1979). Whatever its aetiology, the management of such problems can usually be accomplished rapidly using behavioural techniques (Reading 1982). Other aspects may be more difficult to change. The medical setting may be an unfamiliar and threatening environment, with attempts by nursing staff failing to transcend these difficulties, owing to their dissimilar backgrounds: 'a gap as wide as the River Thames divides the Lambeth mums from the nursing elite with their hockey team accents and unpowdered complexions' (Cohen 1964: p. 27). It is further possible that women smoking heavily or consuming large quantities of alcohol may delay clinic attendance through fear of staff rebuke and/or because they believe themselves unable to alter their behaviour.

Less commonly, women may delay attendance through failure to accept the fact that they are pregnant. Where the pregnancy is unwanted, as in the case of the young unmarried woman living with her parents, the early symptoms of pregnancy may be attributed to other causes. The state of being pregnant may be accepted only at the time of foetal movement, which for a primiparous woman will be around the twentieth week of gestation. A recent Health Education Council poster summarized this concern by stating, 'Don't wait for your baby to prod you into action before going to see the doctor.'

## Smoking

Estimates of the proportion of women who smoke during their pregnancy vary from 42 to 73 per cent. However, the scope of this problem is indicated by statistics on smoking in the population as a whole which indicate that it increased among women, in spite of increasing publicity campaigns to the contrary. For example, between 1969 and 1974 the percentage of regular smokers among females aged between 15 and 16 rose from 9 per cent to 20 per cent and for those aged 17 to 18 from 18 per cent to 25 per cent. Consistent with research showing the deleterious effects of smoking on adult health, evidence is accumulating on its adverse effects in pregnancy. The question to be posed is: if women cannot be stopped from smoking, is it possible to succeed in encouraging them to stop when they realize that their unborn baby's health may be imperilled? Before considering this question, the evidence on the adverse effects of maternal smoking will be examined.

Epidemiological studies have consistently shown that women who smoke have lighter birthweight babies, along with an increased incidence of small-for-dates, prematurity and perinatal mortality (Butler and Goldstein 1973). However, the possibility that smoking women eat less, thereby gaining less weight and therefore giving birth to lighter babies, needs to be entertained. Davies *et al.* (1976) presented evidence to show that mean weekly weight-gain is less if the mother smokes, and that this is reflected in the infant's weight at birth. In order to address the question of the contribution of maternal weight, Meyer (1978) reanalysed the records of the Ontario Perinatal Mortality Study, which collected detailed information on 51,000 births. No significant differences emerged between smokers and non-smokers in terms of low weight-gain. Controlling for maternal weight, there was a clear increase in the proportion of low birthweight babies as the level of maternal smoking increased. Similar findings emerged from a prospective study of over

5,000 Swedish women, of whom 69 per cent were smokers. By repeated ultrasound examination, significant differences were found in the rate of change of foetal biparietal diameter measurements from twenty-eighth week of gestation onwards. These were directly correlated with the number of cigarettes smoked, with reduced foetal growth in women who smoked (Persson *et al.* 1976). Once again, the evidence supported a direct pharmacological effect on the foetus rather than one resulting from nutritional deprivation alone.

The long-term effects of smoking in pregnancy have been also examined. At 6½ years old, children of smoking mothers were found to have more neurological and EEG abnormalities, lower scores on a range of psychological tests and slightly lower school placement than those of non-smoking mothers (Dunn *et al.* 1977). These findings confirm those reported by Butler and Goldstein (1973), who found differences in height, reading, mathematics and general ability at 7 and 11 years.

While a definite conclusion as to causal mechanisms remains to be drawn, smoking during pregnancy has been consistently associated with foetal growth retardation and increased perinatal mortality. The findings from the Ontario Perinatal Mortality Study showed: (a) perinatal mortality was 27 per cent higher in smoking mothers; and (b) the risk of perinatal mortality was increased by 20 per cent when women smoked one pack per day (Fielding 1977). This increased to 35 per cent when smoking in excess of this. Such findings are not altogether surprising when one considers the evidence on the adverse pharmacological effects of tobacco products on the human arteries.

Irrespective of the question of causation, the evidence available offers insights into therapeutic objectives. If the effects of smoking were mediated by low weight-gain on the mother's part, a programme of diet supplementation would be indicated. Alternatively, if smoking constituted a stress-coping response, the treatment choice might be anxiety management techniques. The research gives support to the direct effects of smoking via hypoxia, indicating that the target should be the reduction of smoking itself, possibly combined with nutritional education.

## Alcohol

While the adverse effects of alcohol consumption on the developing foetus were recognized in ancient Greece, with Aristotle observing that drunken women often bore children who were feeble-minded, it is only comparatively recently that the subject has received scientific scrutiny. This is surprising in view of the recognition in England, during the early part of the nineteenth century, of the gin epidemic as an explanation for the decline in population (Coffey 1966). Nevertheless, it was only in the early part of the 1970s that alcohol came to be accorded its deserved role in contributing to antenatal and neonatal problems. By 1977 it had been declared to be one of the 'most frequent known causes of mental deficiency in the Western world' (Clarren and Smith, 1978). Current knowledge suggests that antenatal exposure to alcohol may be associated with a distinct pattern of congenital malformations, referred to as foetal alcohol syndrome (Abel 1980). Among the factors implicated in this syndrome are: intrauterine and postnatal growth deficiency, a distinctive pattern of physical malformation including microcephaly, ocular, facial, joint, limb and cardiac anomalies, and behavioural/cognitive impairment in the form of fine motor dysfunction and mental retardation (Cushner 1981).

The actual number of children affected by alcohol is not known, with estimates of those displaying foetal alcohol syndrome at 1–2 live births per 1,000 (Hanson et al. 1976), with a further 3–5 births per 1,000 exhibiting some features of this syndrome. However, it should be recognized that many such cases pass unrecognized and also that the syndrome may represent the extreme end of a dose response curve in which a positive slope, in terms of adverse effects, begins at a far lower level of alcohol consumption. Thus, safe limits have not yet been established, contrary to earlier pronouncements by such agencies as the US National Institute on Alcohol Abuse and Alcoholism. As drinkers are also likely to be smokers, the additional or synergistic effects of alcohol are of interest and as yet poorly understood.

Two recent studies offer disquieting data to those drinking minimal to moderate amounts. In a survey of 32,000 women, Harlap and Shiono (1980) assessed the combined effects of smoking and alcohol consumption on the incidence of spontaneous abortion in the first two trimesters of pregnancy. Nearly 52 per cent of women were non-drinkers at the first assessment and smoking was reported by 25 per cent, with these behaviours associated. The results showed that regular drinkers, defined as taking one or more drinks per day, had more spontaneous losses, mainly during the second trimester. Other factors emerging as predictive of spontaneous abortion were increased age and parity, race (higher among blacks), previous spontaneous abortions and previous induced abortions among nulliparae. Controlling for these variables, having more than one drink per day remained associated with a higher likelihood of second trimester abortions. Analysis of the relative effects of smoking and drinking indicated these to be independent risk factors, with a greater contribution for drinking than smoking. Kline *et al.* (1980) studied the frequency of alcohol consumption in 616 women who aborted spontaneously and compared this with a control group delivering after at least twenty-eight weeks gestation. In terms of frequency of drinking, 17 per cent of the former group, compared with 8 per cent of controls, admitted drinking twice a week or more. This association remained after controlling for possible confounding variables.

There is evidence to indicate that a combination of smoking and alcohol may have a greater effect on the developing foetus than either alone. For example, Kaminiski et al. (1978) reported an increase in the incidence of stillbirths and lower birthweight among the offspring of women who drank and smoked, compared with women who consumed as much alcohol but did not also smoke. Similarly, Martin et al. (1977) found that infants born to mothers who did both performed less well on learning tasks than did infants born to mothers who either drank or smoked heavily, but not both. In a further report, Martin et al. (1978) reported that infants exposed to both substances *in utero*, as compared with one only, did not suck as hard.

Such studies raise the issue of critical periods of increased risk. Kline et al. (1980) identify the first two trimesters. However, consideration of brain development suggests two periods of heightened vulnerability. The first is between the twelfth and eighteenth weeks of gestation, which is the time of neuronal multiplication. The second occurs during the third trimester and continues over the first eighteen months of life and involves the development of dendritic branching and the formation of synaptic connections (Dobbing 1976). Thus a teratological agent could have maximal effects on the brain and minimal effects on other organs at such times (Abel 1980).

The results of these studies enlarge upon the suggestion that the foetal alcohol syndrome represents the extreme end of a dose response curve (Fielding and Yankauer, 1978). The study by Harlap and Shiono (1980) indicates that alcohol may have deleterious effects not only when abused but also when taken in moderation, once or twice daily. This finding, if replicated, has profound implications for health education campaigns generally, as well as for the information provided in antenatal clinics. The findings of Kline *et al.* (1980) suggest that even less frequent drinking may confer an increased risk of spontaneous abortion. This suggests that the reproductive system may be highly sensitive to alcohol and that spontaneous abortion may be one of the most common manifestations of this sensitivity, the implication being that the newborn with cogenital malformation due to foetal alcohol syndrome may be considered survivors among conceptions heavily exposed to alcohol (Stein *et al.* 1975).

As was seen with cigarette smoking, the consumption of alcohol by females is increasing to achieve parity with men (Bowker 1977). The proportion drinking during pregnancy may be high due, in part, to the relative neglect paid to this by health care professionals. The potential for change may also be high, given that estimates suggest that 94 per cent of women drinkers are social drinkers who do not have an addiction problem (Fielding and Yankauer 1978). However, although to the rational observer pregnancy should constitute a sufficient incentive to give up drinking or smoking, particularly as short-term abstinence is all that is being requested, it is evident that such a viewpoint is overly simplistic.

## Nutrition

The popular expression, 'you are what you eat', acquires an added dimension for the pregnant woman, since nutrition will determine the health and wellbeing of both mother and foetus. Information is available on extreme situations in terms of malnutrition affecting maternal weight-gain, birthweight and the incidence of stillbirth, spontaneous abortion and neonatal health (Worthington 1979). Thus societies in which diet is less ample have a lower average birthweight, with the average in Guatemala and India being 5.5 lbs. However, malnutrition affects only a minority in the Western world; and so we will examine the effects of diet in less extreme circumstances.

Vermeesch (1977) reviewed nutritional supplement programmes during pregnancy and concluded that high-risk mothers can experience more successful pregnancies when superior nutritional guidance is part of their antenatal care. The level of iron ingested is of particular concern, as iron requirments increase during pregnancy and Western diets are commonly relatively low in this compound. As a result many women are prescribed iron supplements early in pregnancy. Folic acid deficiency has been implicated in a range of adverse outcomes. Women at risk of folic acid deficiency, such as those who have been repeatedly pregnant, long-term oral contraceptive users, those who suffer from serious diarrhoea and chronic users of low calorie regimens before pregnancy, may be prescribed a supplement; this has become standard practice in the UK.

The incidence of neural tube defects in the United Kingdom has been consistently greater in women of lower socio-economic status (Williamson 1965). Poor diet in early pregnancy and deficiencies in essential dietary constituents has been suggested as a causal factor (Smithells *et al.* 1976). Laurence *et al.* (1980) studied 176 pregnant women who had a previous child with neural tube defects, and assessed the quality of their diets. Approximately 50 per cent of the sample were provided with additional dietary counselling. They found that 3 of the 109 counselled women and 5 of the 77 in the control condition gave birth to a second child with neural tube defects. All 8 cases had occurred in the 45 women whose diet was considered poor. Of the total number of 18 miscarriages, 15 occurred among the 45 women judged to be taking a poor diet. The authors concluded that improving the quality of the diet, especially during the first trimester of pregnancy, in women at risk of pregnancies complicated by foetal neural tube defects, may improve some environmental factors acting on the foetus. In their study, 58 of the 103 women counselled improved their diets compared with an absence of appropriate change in controls. This study suggests the benefits of systematic counselling for at-risk groups.

## Drugs

In addition to alcohol and smoking, a variety of other drugs are commonly taken during pregnancy. Since almost all compounds have the potential to cross the placenta, the foetus may be exposed to a number of possibly damaging substances. The significance of this problem is indicated by surveys of drugs used during pregnancy. For example, Doering and Stewart (1978) reported an average of eleven different products. The effects of many of these drugs are unknown or inadequately studied, with thalidomide a tragic example of the effects of injudiciously prescribing drugs at this time. In fact, since the majority of drugs are taken for the purpose of alleviating uncomfortable symptoms, not as therapeutic agents, some have questioned their use at all during pregnancy (Forfar and Nelson 1973).

Reliance upon some form of drug as a first line of defence against the problems of modern living may have become such an ingrained habit that many women may not be fully aware of their daily drug intake during pregnancy. A survey of 231 pregnant women revealed that at least one over-the-counter drug was taken by 95 per cent of the women (Hill *et al.* 1977). These included: laxatives, stool softeners, iron preparations, antacids, nasal decongestants, antihistamines, antitussives, antiemetics and sedatives. In addition to those obtained from pharmacists, these women reported also taking tea (75%), coffee

(43%), daily alcohol (7%), cigarettes (23%) and artificial sweeteners (25%). Thirty per cent reported exposure to pesticides, and 28 per cent to paints, solvents, oven cleaners and other chemicals. A more recently recognized problem, possibly more prevalent in the United States than the United Kingdom, is the continued use of marijuana during pregnancy. The US National Institute of Health recently instituted a multicentre study to investigate its effects, thereby acknowledging the importance attached to this behaviour.

Cushner (1981) has considered the question of drug use during pregnancy and remarked: 'Somewhere between the extremes of total license and therapeutic nihilism regarding drug usage and exposure during pregnancy, there must be a rational and realistic approach' (p. 213). This will involve informed decisions by women, necessitating appropriate educational programmes, as well as cautious action or recommendations by the medical practitioner. The evidence indicates both the volume of drugs being used and the possibility that many of these are taken habitually. Simply alerting women to the issues and advising caution may be beneficial.

## Behaviour modification in pregnancy

The evidence reviewed indicates both the variable level of adherence among pregnant women to health advice and the adverse effects on health of failure to comply. The health problem can be considered from a behavioural standpoint, in so far as alterations in behaviour are necessary in order to insure the optimum intrauterine environment for the foetus. While it is possible to identify the need for behavioural change and to recommend that the focus be shifted to education and training in behaviour change, it has to be acknowledged that attempts to promote such change have been less than uniformly successful. Of the factors identified as related to compliance, some are immutable demographic variables, while others are resistant to change (such as patient and doctor attitudes), and others more amenable to modification (drug regimen and clinic management). As a result, the focus of attention in this context has shifted from regarding patients as compliant or noncompliant *per se*, to understanding the patients' perceptions of the medical services (Stimson 1974), and in particular their evaluation of the relevance and value of the help being dispensed (Becker 1974).

## Health beliefs

Evidence suggests that it is insufficient to simply alert patients to the objective seriousness of failing to comply with therapy (Blackwell 1976). Patients with serious conditions fail to comply with drug regimens and smoking is particularly refractory even where smoking-related diseases have been contracted. Little *et al.* (1981) assessed public awareness of risks of drinking in a population survey of telephone subscribers in an area of Oregon in the USA. Comparable proportions of men and women (90 per cent and 85 per cent), nominated drinking and smoking as possibly or definitely harmful to the unborn child. Other than the 13 per cent who felt women should abstain altogether from alcohol, the majority believed an unsafe level to be more than 2 to 3 drinks daily. Men recommended significantly higher 'safe' levels than women and those respondents who themselves drank or smoked evinced generally more liberal attitudes. The main conclusion to be drawn from this study is not new but worth restating. The data indicate that awareness of risk is no guarantee that appropriate action will follow to reduce that risk. Additional techniques of behavioural management may be needed in order to translate awareness into action. Similarly, Graham (1976) studied the attitudes of fifty smoking women to their behaviour in the face of health advice to refrain. Those smoking displayed acceptance or rejection of the evidence, with the former experiencing feelings of inadequacy and guilt. This study illustrates the dilemma of health educators, as it showed not that ignorance was operating but rather that what was important was the credibility attached to this information.

The health belief model (Becker 1974) represents an attempt to describe behaviour and decision-making under conditions of uncertainty. It suggests that behaviour can be predicted from both the individual's evaluation of an outcome and the expectation that a specific action will result in that outcome consisting of: (a) the motivation to avoid an illness or to become well; (b) the amount of desire for a particular level of health; (c) the belief that a specific health action will prevent or ameliorate illness. The model also postulates the need for a relevant stimulus or cue to action which must occur to trigger the appropriate health behaviour; this stimulus may be internal or external (Becker 1976). It is informative to consider pregnancy from this conceptual framework. Cues for action can be seen at two levels (i) becoming pregnant itself may enhance the relevance of health advice; and (ii) contact with the foetus, via foetal movement perception or by feedback via ultrasound, may also act to facilitate appropriate behavioural changes. The former suggests that pregnancy may be a fruitful stage at which to provide preventive health advice, since the likelihood of behavioural change may be higher. The potential of heightened foetal awareness in promoting change has been considered in a report of health behaviour in women provided with different levels of feedback via ultrasound. Women seeing the foetus reported more appropriate change in smoking and alcohol consumption over the subsequent four weeks than those not viewing the monitor screen (Reading *et al.* 1982a).

In addition to educational efforts designed to raise women's awareness of possible risks, it is necessary to offer specific techniques to facilitate behaviour change. For many women, simply recognizing the relevance of the information and the need to change will be sufficient to achieve the desired result. Where the problem is longstanding, specific therapy programmes will be called for, designed to break the habits of smoking or drinking and to substitute appropriate and competing activities.

To date, little systematic work has been carried out. The available data are not very encouraging about the benefits of such programmes. Donovan (1977) reported that the effects of intensive individual antismoking counselling were comparable to standard care, which included anti-smoking education. However, education may be supplemented with techniques derived from behaviour modification programmes with habit disorders. One such technique, that of rapid smoking, was evaluated by Danaher *et al.* (1978). Of the 11 women enrolled in the programme, 3 discontinued, with the remaining 8 reporting reduced levels.

## Conclusion and implications

Although there have been dramatic improvements in perinatal mortality rates over the last thirty years, a number of problems remain. As has been shown in this chapter, the health of the pregnant woman, and her foetus by implication, may be greatly influenced by what she does, or does not do, during the gestational period. Sufficient evidence has been collected to implicate smoking and alcohol in the cause of perinatal problems, with nutrition and drug use other areas of concern. It would be reasonable to expect that a significant reduction in the number of pregnant women who use alcohol, tobacco and drugs would contribute to a reduction in the number of low birthweight infants and the number of birth defects. However, the return on investment of resources to eliminate these risks completely (which is probably impossible) remains unclear, since women who smoke and drink are very often also at risk for other reasons. However, continued efforts to promote appropriate health behaviour during pregnancy can be seen as worthwhile when the perspective is broadened to include the woman's subsequent health and the outcome of subsequent pregnancies.

In conclusion, intervention during pregnancy should recognize the following:

1. that risk behaviours are highly correlated. This would avoid the isolationist approach of focusing only on smoking or drinking;
2. that pregnancy may be a time of optimum receptivity for behavioural change and that attempts should be made to encourage mothers to maintain the gains made during pregnancy after the birth;
3. that education alone may be insufficient in all cases and that women should be offered additional help by drawing on behaviour modification techniques;
4. that pregnancy represents a time of extended contact with the health profession for both the woman and her family, and offers an opportunity to disseminate preventive health care information.

Whether antenatal health care services respond to such challenges remains to be seen.

## Chapter 4

# The evolution of maternal feelings

Having considered the adverse effects of anxiety and certain behaviour during pregnancy, it is time to reflect upon the development of maternal feelings. Assuming initially ambivalent attitudes towards the pregnancy, what factors facilitate positive attitude change during pregnancy? In particular, interest will be focused on the interplay between psychological state, in terms of the onset of maternal feelings, and physical changes of both negative and positive valency. Many of the themes to be introduced will be further developed in Chapter 7 on bonding, since the focus on the postpartum period for the development of the mother-neonate bond has obscured the significance of the antenatal period in preparing the woman for interaction with her neonate. Two assumptions will be made: (a) that what happens during pregnancy will affect initial reactions to the neonate, since pre-existing negative attitudes are unlikely to dissipate completely upon seeing the newborn; (b) that many women initially experience ambivalent or negative attitudes, indicating the importance of understanding factors facilitating positive attitudes change. The second assumption follows from viewing the occasion of conception as a time of both loss and gain. For some the loss of an old identity may be the predominant attitude, while for others doubts are obscured by the eager anticipation of motherhood. It is not surprising that women describe emotions ranging from delight to despair upon confirmation of pregnancy.

## The crisis of pregnancy

The early view of pregnancy as a partly dream-like period, fulfilling a woman's deepest yearnings (Deutsch 1943), has largely been superseded by recognition of it as one of the major female transition points or developmental crises (Bibring 1959). Although it has become accepted that women may typically feel ambivalence or a degree of negativity during the initial states of gestation, these feelings are believed to diminish once foetal movement has become established. Such normative values are important as they create the conditions for strain in those cases where the woman fails to experience the feelings expected of her. Where negative attitudes persist, these have been related to the absence of close social support, poor relationship with their own mother and a tendency for neurotic symptoms to be present. With the greater tolerance in attitudes over the past years, it has become further recognized that ambivalence may be expressed in ways other than outright rejection. The occurrence of emotional disturbance, in the form of depression, irritability, anxiety and fears may be indicative of adjustment difficulties, as might the persistence of physical symptoms. An indication of the myopic approach of theorists in this field concerns the implicit assumption that conflicts become resolved following the birth. Social surveys have documented the continuing stress imposed on both the woman and the marriage in a proportion of cases (Wolkind and Zajicek 1981).

## Nausea and vomiting

In addition to attitudinal changes, pregnancy involves many physical changes and complaints, such as painful and swollen breasts, nausea and morning sickness, tiredness, lassitude, and uncustomary food cravings. The degree to which pronounced physical symptoms reflect difficulties in adjusting to the pregnancy has been the subject of many studies. Nausea and vomiting have attracted a great deal of attention in this respect. Psychoanalytic thought has provided two competing explanations for the presence or absence of this symptom. The most commonly held view is that these symptoms are a manifestation of an unconscious desire not to be pregnant, with the vomiting seen as a symbolic means of expressing this desire. The symptoms are thought to subside with the advent of foetal movement because at this time the woman is confronted with the reality of the autonomous existence of the foetus, so that it cannot be 'thrown up', and comes to adjust to the pregnancy. An alternative view is that the symptom-free pregnancy should be viewed with suspicion as suggestive of the woman's denial of her condition.

The causes of nausea and vomiting in pregnancy are unknown. Although there appears to be a firm physiological basis to this symptom (with human chorionic gonadotrophin instrumental), questions remain as to the reasons for the variation in occurrence and persistence. Estimates suggest it occurs in between 50 per cent and 75 per cent of gravid women. It has been regarded as a favourable prognostic sign; for women carrying a single foetus, the risk of abortion prior to the twentieth week is thought to be less if nausea is present. Similarly, liveborn children are reported to be of greater gestational age and higher birthweight than children born to women in whom these symptoms are absent (Brandes 1967). The protective value of these symptoms may derive from their causing the woman to restrict her activities, thereby increasing the likelihood of survival of a vulnerable foetus.

A question of interest which has attracted research attention is why nausea occurs in only a proportion of pregnant women. Coppen (1959) investigated a random sample of 50 pregnant women, 29 of whom had suffered from these symptoms. No differences emerged between the two groups on a range of measures which included psychiatric histories, mental state, sexual functioning, attitude to pregnancy and their experience of stressful events. Other studies have related the symptoms to psychological adjustment during pregnancy. Uddenberg *et al.* (1971) studied 152 Swedish women and detected differences between women reporting no symptoms, severe symptoms or mild problems. Those declaring severe or no problems were more likely to have psychiatric symptoms before or during the pregnancy. Similarly, women in the mild group were more likely to have planned their pregnancy.

A sample of London women was studied by Wolkind and Zajicek (1981). Those women who complained of prolonged vomiting could be distinguished by the general lack of support they received. In particular, their husbands were less involved in preparing for the arrival of the first child. Women showing a good adjustment to the pregnancy were also likely to display the symptom of nausea. This should not be taken to suggest that poor adjustment may be the case in the absence of the symptom. No support was found for the viewpoint that the nausea represents a rejection of the foetus. They do suggest that sickness extending beyond the first trimester may indicate the need for a fuller psychosocial evaluation; that this symptom may constitute a cry for help.

By way of serendipitous findings, Little and Hook (1979) found that women who admitted to being regular smokers and drinkers experienced less nausea and vomiting. This raises the reverse possibility that women experiencing fewer of these symptoms may be smokers or drinkers. Data becoming available on the effects of marijuana use in pregnancy, have found less use of antiemetics in women admitting to regular marijuana use. These findings are hardly surprising when we consider the current clinical trials of marijuana use in cancer treatment for the control of chemotherapy side-effects, owing to its established antiemetic action (Ungerleider *et al.* 1981).

## The impact of quickening

Turning to sensations more often accompanied by positive feelings, what are the psychological effects of foetal movement sensations? Klaus and Kennell (1976), best known for their work on maternal-infant bonding, have considered the nature of attitude changes over the course of pregnancy. They have identified a number of events as important in the evolution of maternal feelings, among which are: planning the pregnancy, confirming the pregnancy, foetal movement perception and seeing the baby. It is the experience of foetal movement sensation, or quickening, which has been identified as important in preparing the woman for the birth and the physical separation from the child, because through it she is made aware of the autonomous nature of the foetus. It is noteworthy that foetal movement only becomes established as the likelihood of spontaneous abortion diminishes. Such changes are shown schematically in Fig. 2. There is a noticeable increase in 'investment in the foetus' contingent upon foetal movement perception. Investment in the foetus is believed to be reflected in active, practical preparations for the new baby, commonly referred to as 'nesting'. Although such changes will have behavioural manifestations, and so be amenable to empirical study,

## 48  Psychological aspects of pregnancy

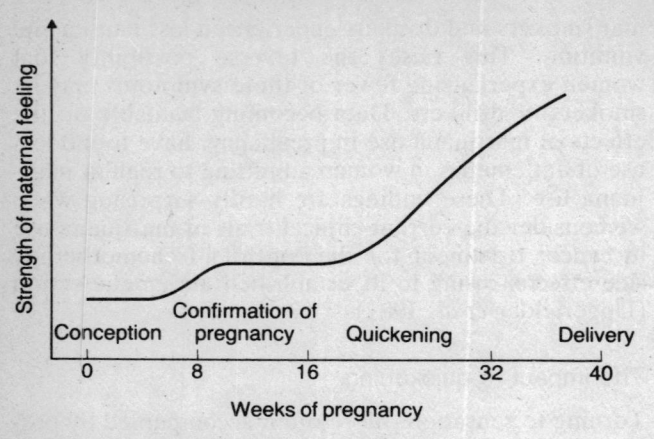

*Fig. 2*  The evolution of maternal feelings

there have been few attempts to document the role of quickening in precipitating these, or in establishing the degree to which women display a uniform pattern of attitudinal change. As was seen in Chapter 3, attitudes towards the pregnancy and the prospect of motherhood may mediate behavioural changes necessary to insure the optimum intrauterine environment for the foetus, in terms of stopping smoking and avoiding alcohol and other drugs.

Maternal monitoring of foetal movement is acknowledged to be a valuable and relatively simple technique for following the health of the foetus during the last trimester. Maternal awareness of decreased foetal activity is a sign of foetal hypoxia. With the use of objective recording of foetal movement by ultrasound, it is now possible to assess the accuracy with which women are able to perceive foetal activity. Such surveys have confirmed the sensitivity and consistency of the majority of women in reporting foetal movement (Hertogs *et al.* 1979). However, a small number of women are relatively insensitive to such movements. It has been speculated that sensitivity may be related to acceptance of the pregnancy, although no empirical test of such a proposition has been made yet.

## Ultrasonic feedback of foetal movement

The increasing use of ultrasound in antenatal care is relevant to an understanding of attitude changes during pregnancy, since with the advent of real-time ultrasound women may be now exposed to moving images of their foetus *in utero*. The psychological implications of foetal diagnostic procedures will be considered in greater detail in the following chapter. For present purposes, the focus will be on the psychological effects of early exposure. It is possible that ultrasound feedback of the foetus *in utero*, early in the second trimester of pregnancy, may have analogous effects to, and anticipate and augment, the awareness brought on by foetal movement perception. This feedback of internal physiological events, otherwise beyond conscious awareness, may result in changes comparable to those believed to occur with quickening. Studies of the psychological effects of ultrasound have reported uniformly positive reactions (Kohn *et al*. 1980; Milne *et al*. 1981) with more uniformly positive attitudes towards the pregnancy and the foetus reported following an ultrasound examination (Campbell *et al*. 1982). By providing direct feedback early in the pregnancy, ultrasound may facilitate the emotional and attitudinal changes necessary to bring about adaptive behaviour change. Anxiety over the viability of the pregnancy may be reduced by ultrasound confirmation of foetal movement and development. Similarly, increased awareness of the foetus *in utero* may promote adherence to antenatal health care advice by enhancing the perceived relevance and salience of this information (Reading *et al*. 1982a). Since ultrasound feedback is feasible some weeks prior to the onset of quickening, there may be greater potential for benefit to the foetus, through earlier avoidance by the woman of smoking or alcohol.

## Sexual behaviour

Sexuality during pregnancy is relevant to this discussion, since sexual feelings and behaviour may be affected by increased awareness of the foetus. Moreover, couples are understandably concerned as to the implications of various forms of sexual practice for the foetus and pregnancy. Unfortunately, this issue has received comparatively little attention in the literature and may not be included in routine antenatal interviews. The evidence suggests that it is important to determine whether a woman is sexually active and to provide an opportunity for questions and concerns to be raised. Evidence on doctor-patient communication demonstrates the importance of good doctor/patient interaction in dealing with this topic. Where patients perceive doctors to be ill-at-ease they may be disinclined to raise sexual difficulties, even though such problems may have been the only reason for seeking the consultation.

One of the first empirical studies on this topic was conducted by Masters and Johnson (1966), who reported an initial decrease in coital frequency and desire during the first trimester, followed by an increase during the second. The third trimester was marked by a fall in both interest and activity. More recently, Solberg *et al.* (1973) documented a steady decline in sexual activity over the entire course of the pregnancy. They also reported a decrease in frequency of orgasm by intercourse and a diminished level of sexual intensity. Orgasm through manual stimulation by the partner was not affected, although masturbation frequency declined. Only 15 per cent of the sample of

260 had received specific advice from the obstetrician. A change in preferred coital position was reported, with decreased use of the male superior method. The reasons given for diminished sexual interest were: physical discomfort (46%), fear of injury to the baby (27%), loss of interest in sex (23%), awkwardness while having sex (17%), compliance with obstetric recommendation (8%), extraneous reasons (8%), loss of attractiveness on woman's part (6%), recommendation of friend (1%) and unspecified (15%). Of the sample, 29 per cent received specific instructions from their doctor to abstain for between 2 and 8 weeks before their estimated date of confinement.

The data suggest a decline in sexuality during pregnancy, although they are of little help in unravelling the contributions of hormonal, metabolic and physical factors. One of the major reasons cited for discontinuing intercourse is fear of harm to the foetus, by causing infection or stimulating uterine contractions. There appears to be little evidence to suggest that damage may be caused by the penis during coital thrusting, in the absence of pre-existing bleeding, ruptured membranes or threatened premature labour. Infection may be a threat where the cervix and membranes are providing inadequate protection, as when the cervix dilates or the membranes rupture. The evidence suggests that orgasm, rather than the act of penetration, is capable of stimulating uterine contractions. Goodlin (1973) presented case material in support of this: 4 out of 5 women achieved orgasm at term, following which 3 commenced labour and the fourth a false labour. Similarly, Wagner *et al.* (1976) observed an association between prematurity and multiple orgasm during pregnancy in 19 women, with a number recollecting the onset of contractions following intercourse.

If these observations are confirmed, what are the mechanisms of action? It is known that uterine contractions occur during orgasm. Fox and Knaggs (1969) were able to detect the presence of oxytocin in blood samples taken one minute after female orgasm. Oxytocin is used to induce labour and so its endogenous release via orgasm may serve an analagous function. A more speculative explanation concerns the presence of prostaglandins in seminal fluid. Prostaglandins are known to be associated with uterine contractions and are also used to induce labour.

These surveys raise a number of issues. Offering couples information on what is known about sexual functioning in pregnancy may be helpful. The potential hazards of orgasm close to term can be described. It is interesting that a survey on behaviour matched to preferences identified a preference for less sex than was occurring during the third trimester, but a need for more physical affection and closeness (Tolor and DiGrazia 1976). Supplying accurate information may assist couples to achieve a balance between gratifying their needs and safeguarding the foetus.

## Conclusion

It is evident that little systematic research has been conducted on the nature of emotional changes during pregnancy. Theories emphasize the importance of physical change in facilitating attitude change and instigating appropriate self-care behaviour. This would be amenable to empirical tests. The way in which awareness of the foetus influences sexual feelings and behaviour is also of interest.

Chapter 5

# Antenatal foetal diagnosis: the woman's perspective

## Introduction

There has been intensive research in recent years on the development of methods for the antenatal diagnosis of congenital conditions and the identification of foetal abnormalities. If this can be accomplished before twenty weeks gestation, couples may be offered the option of selective abortion of the affected foetus. The expansion of these services, with an increasing number of women undergoing these procedures, raises a number of psychological issues, which will be discussed in this chapter. Before doing so, the nature of the diagnostic techniques currently available will be briefly described.

## Diagnostic procedures

There are three main methods of detecting foetal anomalies and abnormalities: amniocentesis, foetoscopy and ultrasound. Amniocentesis, which involves withdrawing a sample of the uterine amniotic fluid, was the first to become available. The diagnosis of genetic defects in the foetus is possible by cytological and biochemical analysis of the amniotic fluid in order to detect chromosomal aberrations, such as those responsible for Down's syndrome. Since this procedure is invasive, it carries a low risk of miscarriage. Analysis of the amniotic fluid may also provide information on the level of alpha-foetoprotein (AFP), which is raised in the presence of open neural-tube defects such as spina bifida, anencephaly, hydrocephaly, microcephaly and encephalocele. Foetoscopy permits examination of external foetal structures by direct visualization. This means that very small anatomical structures such as hands, feet and genitalia are clearly visualized. Its disadvantage is the increased risk of subsequent abortion, estimated at between 3 per cent and 6 per cent (Rodeck and Campbell 1979). It is used where there is a suspicion of a small external defect which is beyond the resolving power of ultrasound and which cannot be diagnosed by biochemical analysis of the amniotic fluid.

The third technique, ultrasound, may be used in conjunction with the former two, or by itself. Ultrasound consists of transmitting very sharp pulses (in the region of 1 $\mu$ sec) of high frequency, low-intensity soundwaves through the woman's abdomen. Because the duty cycle is long, the acoustic power of the system is extremely low and well within all known safety margins (Hobbins *et al.* 1979). The soundwave passes down through maternal and foetal tissues, being gradually attenuated in the process. The reflected soundwaves are converted into electric signals which are then amplified and processed by cathode ray tube into visual signals. There are two basic ultrasound modalities used in foetal visualization: static B scanning and real-time scanning. The former produces high resolution static pictures. By making multiple two-diminsional longitudinal or cross-sectional 'slices' of the foetus, the operator is able to construct a three-dimensional image of the foetus. This is the optimal modality for making the diagnosis of foetal abnormality. Its disadvantages

## Antenatal foetal diagnosis 55

are the high costs and skills involved and the time required to complete a scan.

Real-time scanning provides a moving image of the foetus and its advantage is that equipment is small and portable. Ultrasound may be used to (1) enhance the safety and effectiveness of amniocentesis, (2) diagnose multiple pregnancy, (3) accurately define foetal age, (4) detect abnormalities in foetal growth rate, (5) detect changes in amniotic fluid volume, and (6) directly detect foetal structural abnormalities (Campbell 1980).

### Psychological impact

Our concern here is not so much the mechanics of this technology but its psychological effects. There has been considerable controversy surrounding the expansion of technology in antenatal and obstetric care. As mortality rates decline so morbidity may increase, through the dehumanizing effects of such technology. Many obstetric units are becoming more like laboratories or computer terminals than settings in which the traditional bedside manner may prevail. Of special concern is the way in which the focus may shift from interaction with patients to a preoccupation with the technology. This has certainly been a valid argument in other medical specialities, where patient contact and time spent interacting with the patient have decreased as technological demands on staff time have increased.

While the diagnostic benefits of these procedures in obstetrics may have been established, comparatively little attention has been given to their psychological impact, other than in the context of concern over this increasing mechanization of obstetric services. Research in other medical settings indicates that such procedures, however benign they may appear, can give rise to concern. There have been suggestions in the literature and the popular press that high technology obstetrics is introducing its own set of problems. As a result, some women are becoming vehemently opposed to the use of such techniques. Rather than enter this debate, it is proposed to review the evidence on the psychological effects of undergoing amniocentesis and ultrasound. In addition to those women who refuse to undergo these procedures it is evident that a number are failing to utilize facilities through lack of awareness of their purpose. Acceptability of methods of assessing foetal wellbeing will be considered, since these raise moral, religious and ethical issues. Acceptance of those procedures carries with it the implication of terminating the pregnancy should an abnormality be identified, which may be an unacceptable option for a proportion of women.

## Psychological effects of amiocentesis

Comparatively little information is available on the subjective perceptions of women toward amniocentesis, or on their reactions to having to undergo this procedure, as compared with the literature on rates of use and the nature of abnormalities found. Chervin *et al.* (1977) sent questionnaires to 67 women at the time they received the results of the amniotic tap and 31 were returned. Several complaints were registered about the 'disturbing' atmosphere of the clinic where the amniocentesis had been performed. Uniformly positive comments were made about the pre-amniocentesis counselling, with 17 of the responses rated as displaying high accuracy of information recalled. A bipolar distribution emerged with respect to pain and discomfort, with over half rating this as insignificant and 7 severe. Most admitted to high anxiety following the procedure. The length of time involved was the most common complaint, since there is a delay of up to four weeks from the time of the procedure to knowing the results. Of this sample, 29 stated they would undergo the procedure again in a subsequent pregnancy.

A comparable study was reported by Dixson *et al.* (1981) in which, in addition to studying 53 women electing to undergo amniocentesis, a control group of 22 women declining this were also studied. The majority of women in both groups had been offered the procedure because of high maternal age, with none at high risk of chromosomal abnormality. Only a third had first heard of the service through the media, suggesting a need for public education in this area. The factors most affecting the control group's decision not to proceed with an amniocentesis were fear of foetal injury, fear of miscarriage and religious beliefs. A difference emerged between the groups as to the anticipated impact of having a defective baby, with one-half of those undergoing amniocentesis believing this would have a substantial impact, as compared with one-quarter of the control group. It is interesting that 25 per cent of the women in both groups continued to be concerned about the outcome of the pregnancy. In terms of reactions to the procedure itself, most felt it had been as, or less difficult than, expected, with once again the most difficult aspect being the waiting period. Interestingly, more than 50 per cent believed their feelings of attachment to the baby had increased during the waiting period. Regarding the decision to be made if the test results were abnormal, while 63 per cent of controls felt they could not have terminated such a pregnancy, only 7 per cent of the women accepting this procedure believed this would not have been possible. No abnormalities were detected by amniocentesis and the only abnormality at birth (neural tube defect) involved a woman declining to undergo this procedure.

A study by Blumberg *et al.* (1975) examined the psychological sequelae of abortion performed for a genetic indication. They studied fifteen families undergoing therapeutic abortion. The most notable finding was that of depression. Such abortions differ in two important respects from elective terminations: they occur later in pregnancy, affording the opportunity for the mother to become more attached to the foetus, especially if quickening has been established; and these women want their pregnancy to be viable and it is usually planned. The procedure involved in later terminations may be intrinsically more distressing than those conducted between 8 and 12 weeks gestation. Once again, the authors identified the four week waiting period for the results of the amniocentesis as a time of particular family strain.

## Acceptability of amniocentesis

The preceding research has been concerned with the reactions of women undergoing amniocentesis. In parallel to this, studies have examined the perceptions and attitudes of pregnant and non-pregnant women to the genetic counselling and diagnostic services in general. This research attention derives from the realization that a substantial proportion of pregnant women are not utilizing the genetic counselling services, with indications that this may be more pronounced in certain segments of the population, those of minority ethnic status or low socio-economic status. While it needs to be acknowledged that this may constitute a rational decision for a proportion of women, in accordance with moral or religious beliefs, for others it may reflect insufficient knowledge, irrational fears or a failure to have assimilated information on availability. The goal of genetic counselling programmes would be to enable couples to achieve informed decisions about conception and future pregnancies, by ensuring that services are seen to be both accessible and acceptable.

While recognition of amniocentesis as a safe procedure has been accompanied by an exponential rise in the number carried out, the greatest use of these services has been by patients with higher incomes and greater educational achievement (Golbus *et al.*, 1979). As an index of access and acceptability, the rate of antenatal diagnosis among women over thirty-five years old has been compared across six states in the USA (Adams *et al.* 1981). The computed utilization ratio varied widely between states. However, a consistent finding was that older women (those over 40) did not have higher utilization ratios, in spite of being at greater risk. Rural areas had lower ratios than urban areas. It is encouraging that use ratios improved between 1977 and 1978, with two states showing an increase of 40 per cent.

Further information is supplied by surveys of users and non-users at particular clinics. Marion *et al.* (1980) presented data on the accessibility of genetic services to low-income patients in Atlanta, Georgia. Of 522 patients counselled, 157 were offered amniocentesis and 61 per cent accepted. For most of the 157, age was the indication for referral and of those only 5 per cent had any prior knowledge of genetic risk. Over this time period, 188 patients of over 35 years who initiated antenatal care too late for antenatal diagnosis were interviewed, of whom 54 per cent declared they would have accepted this procedure had it been feasible. Of those recommended for amniocentesis, 21 declined on religious grounds and 13 through fear of undergoing the procedure. The authors pointed out that the overall utilization rate of amniocentesis among all patients 35 years and older was only 17 per cent. Two factors were predictive of this: delay in seeking antenatal care and poor awareness of increased genetic risk. Similarly, Wilson *et al.* (1979) reported a non-acceptance rate of 27 per cent out of 1,099 women referred to the

University of Southern California Hospital. The most commonly reported reasons for this decision were: 1) concern about the safety of the procedure; 2) antenatal anxiety alleviated by counselling alone; 3) spontaneous abortion; 4) elected medical abortion without the amniocentesis; 5) an erroneous diagnosis of pregnancy; 6) pregnancy too far advanced; 7) patient preferred not to know.

These figures suggest that access is improving but that for a proportion of pregnant women genetic services remain elusive. That a number will refuse to undergo amniocentesis has consistently been found. Where this is related to fears or irrational beliefs, careful counselling and information may ensure that an informed decision is being taken. A number will find the prospect of therapeutic abortion unacceptable. A further problem, which has already been commented upon in Chapter 3, is the proportion who are ineligible owing to their late initial attendance for antenatal care.

The studies on psychological reactions to the procedure itself suggest the need for detailed preparatory counselling to ensure awareness of the delay period. It is customary practice in many clinics to resolve anxieties about harming the foetus by showing the woman her foetus via ultrasound upon completion of the tap. While this may allay anxiety, it may promote the attachment process which has been reported to occur during the time spent waiting for the results. The effect of this on the psychological adjustment to a subsequent therapeutic termination introduces the question of the psychological reactions to ultrasonography, which will be considered next.

## Psychological reactions to ultrasound

With the advent of ultrasonography, many women now undergo scans during pregnancy on one or many occasions. With the development of small and portable real-time scanners, the possibility has emerged of routinely screening the entire antenatal population early in the second trimester. This would accomplish three objectives: to detect certain foetal anomalies, to diagnose multiple pregnancy and to determine foetal age accurately. For example, at King's College Hospital, London, women routinely receive three scans during their pregnancy. These occur at the time of their first antenatal clinic visit, when they undergo a real-time scan; followed by a B-scan at 16 weeks and a further B scan at 32 weeks gestation. In the event of a problem arising, they may receive additional scans in accordance with clinical requirements.

Real-time ultrasound provides two-dimensional pictures of the foetus, with movement visible if the foetus is active at the time of recording. If the monitor is visible to the woman, she may be exposed to pictures of her foetus *in utero*. Similarly, if the partner attends, it may be possible for him to view the foetus. Some units provide parents with a polaroid picture of their foetus so that they are now able to include pictures of the foetus in their photograph albums. The psychological effects of seeing the foetus, and of this technology in general, are once again of interest. To critics of technology this represents a further extension of the alienating effects of such procedures, believed to disrupt the natural processes occurring during the pregnancy. Of particular interest are the effects of early exposure to ultrasound feedback, as women are now able to see their foetus before experiencing foetal movement, which hitherto has been considered to be the first direct contact between mother and foetus and so heralds the confirmation of the pregnancy. Unsystematic observations of women in antenatal clinics where scanning is performed suggest a positive reaction to ultrasound, in that women commonly express delight at seeing the foetus and declare their intention to take better care of themselves. Similar reactions have been confirmed in two nursing studies. Kohn *et al.* (1980) assessed the reactions of 100 primigravidae before and after ultrasonography. Mothers were uniformly positive, with the awareness of foetal movement particularly exciting for those who had not experienced quickening. Similarly, Milne and Rich (1981), studying 30 women in the second and third trimesters, reported positive reactions, raising the possibility that scanning increases the woman's attachment to the foetus.

## Ultrasound: a controlled study

The psychological effects of ultrasound have been subjected to systematic study (Campbell *et al.* 1982). It was intended to evaluate the short- and long-term effects of ultrasound on attitudes and behaviour, by manipulating the level of information or feedback supplied to the woman at the time of her first scan. Women included in the study could be considered a low-risk population, since the aim was to document the effects in this population before proceeding to study at-risk groups, even though it is acknowledged that it is with the latter that ultrasound may have most relevance or impact from a psychological standpoint. Therefore, only women between 18 and 32, in a stable relationship and Caucasian were included. Those with a previous history of miscarriage or who had undergone extended infertility treatment were excluded along with those identified by accredited criteria as at risk of congenital malformation. Women meeting these study criteria were randomly assigned at the first clinic visit to two ultrasound conditions, with a no-scan control group introduced during the course of recruitment. The design is shown in Fig. 3 and indicates that one-half of the sample were shown the monitor screen and received specific visual and verbal feedback as to

```
                Random assignment
                  of primiparae ────────────────┐
                         │                       │
                         │                       │
                  Pre-assessment                 │
                    ╱         ╲                  │
                   ╱           ╲                 │
          High feedback    Low feedback     Control
           ultrasound      ultrasound      condition
                                          (no ultrasound)
                │               │              │
        ┌───────┴───────────────┴──────────────┴───────┐
        │              Post-assessment                 │
        └──────────────────────────────────────────────┘
                                                       │
                                                       ▼
                                                   Ultrasound
```

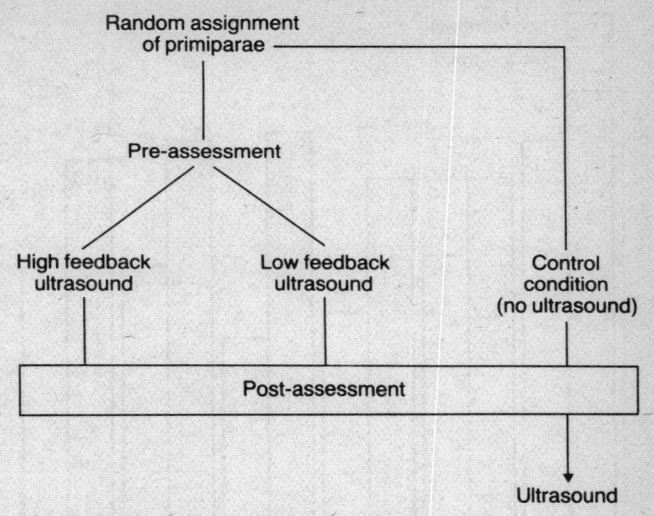

*Fig. 3* Experimental design of the ultrasound study

foetal size, shape and movement. The remainder received a comparable examination with one exception – the monitor screen was turned to one side so that it was not visible to the woman being scanned. These women received only global feedback of the form 'all is well'.

Comparisons were made between the two groups in terms of attitudes towards both the foetus and being pregnant, before and after the ultrasound examination. They were also asked to describe their emotional state at the time and to rate their attitudes towards the procedure. The results showed that women in both ultrasound conditions displayed more uniformly positive attitudes, towards both the pregnancy and the foetus, following the scan. Between-group differences emerged for emotional state and attitudes towards the procedure. As can be seen from Fig. 4, women in the

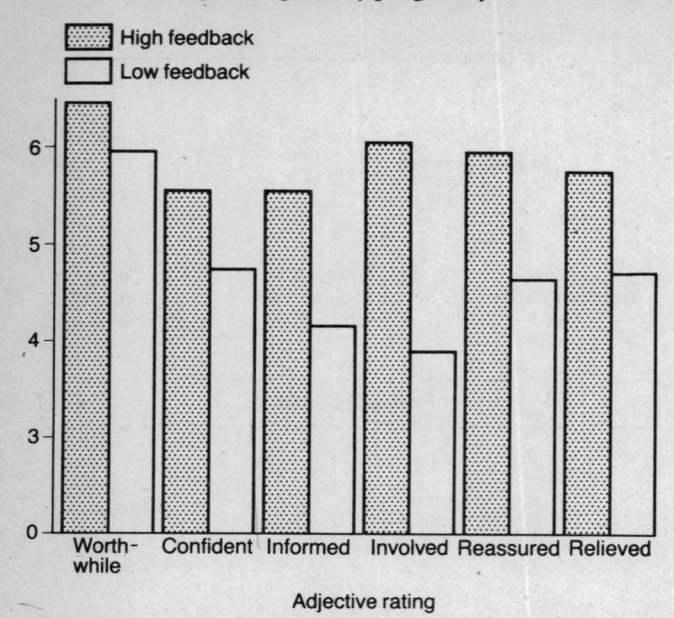

*Fig. 4* Post-scan attitude ratings

high feedback condition, those seeing the monitor screen, reported themselves to be significantly more confident, informed, involved, reassured and relieved, and the procedure as more worthwhile. They also expressed less uncertainty, with scores relating to discomfort and distress uniformly low, attesting to the acceptability of this procedure. Subjective reports of emotional state during the examination are displayed in Fig. 5. Considerable consensus emerged for the high feedback condition with respect to the adjective chosen, with over 70 per cent declaring their emotional state during the scan as 'wonderful!'

Further assessments over the course of the pregnancy and following delivery confirmed the positive

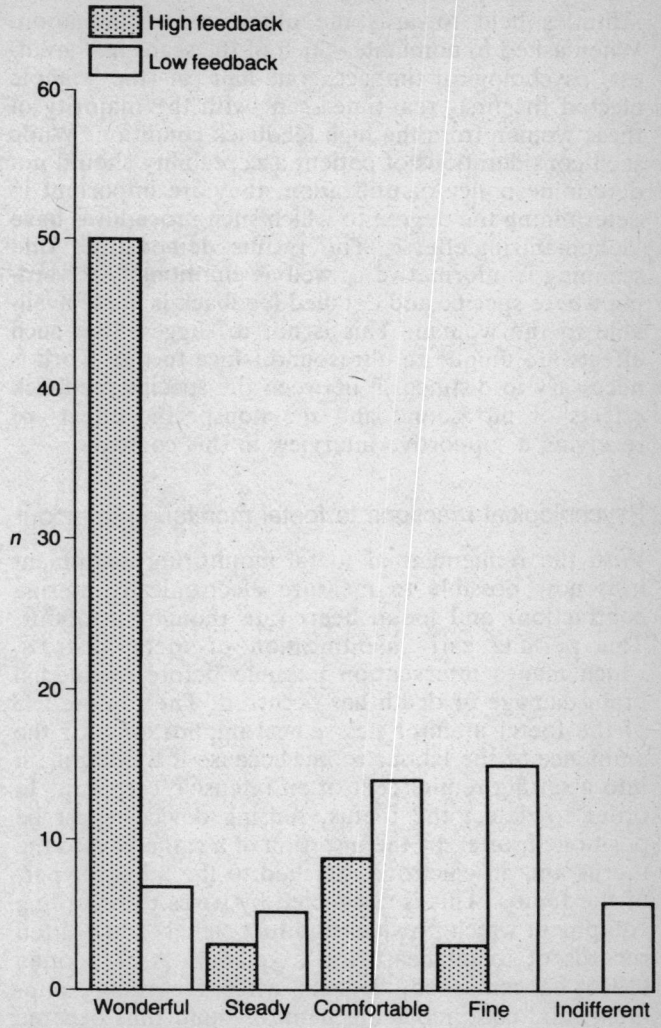

*Fig. 5* Distribution of adjective choices from the subjective stress scale

attitudes held towards the ultrasound examination. When asked to nominate which of the scans had greatest psychological impact, one-half of the sample elected the first, real-time scan, with the majority of these women from the high feedback condition. While such considerations of patient acceptability should not determine policy or utilization, they are important in determining the degree to which such procedures have 'dehumanizing' effects. The results demonstrate that scanning is informative as well as emotionally rewarding where specific and detailed feedback is made available to the woman. This is not to suggest that such effects are unique to ultrasound, since further work is necessary to distinguish between the specific feedback effects of ultrasound and the nonspecific effects of receiving a supportive interview in this context.

## Psychological reactions to foetal monitoring in labour

With the refinement of foetal monitoring equipment it is now possible to measure electronically uterine contractions and foetal heart rate thoughout labour. This permits early identification of foetal distress, which makes intervention possible before irremedial brain damage or death has occurred. The routine use of the foetal monitor has radical implications for the ambience of the labour room, because it transforms it into a setting reminiscent of an intensive care unit. In order to detect the foetus, sensing devices must be positioned, often by the insertion of a catheter into the uterus and an electrode attached to the adjacent part of the foetus. This is connected by wires to recording equipment which provides auditory signals and written records of foetal heart-rate frequency. As Starkman (1976) has remarked, 'Sensors, wires, recording equipment, and continuous mechanical sound thus become prominent features in the environment and experience of both physician and patient.' Starkman (1976) went on to present the results of interviewing twenty-five women in order to elicit reactions to the foetal monitor. A variety of responses were evident, with the monitor seen as a protector of foetal well-being, a means of telling the doctor what was happening, obtaining direct feedback of foetal wellbeing, facilitating the involvement of the husband and a distraction. Negative responses concerned the way in which patient and monitor competed for attention, the increased physical discomfort, the enforced immobility and concern about injury to the foetus. Those women expressing greatest dissatisfaction were those who had a previous experience of uncomplicated labours and health, as well as previous liveborn infants. For these women the equipment was seen as intrusive and an obstacle to being able to realize their anticipated labour course.

An analogy has been drawn between the use of technology in labour and the stress imposed by monitoring devices in intensive care units, in particular coronary care units. The latter have been associated with a variety of adverse psychological reactions, since such environments may have much in common with those producing sensory deprivation experiences. Childbirth differs from cardiac monitoring in a number of important respects. It is the culmination of a period of planned and welcome anticipation and not the sequel to a sudden and calamitous illness. Similarly, cardiac monitoring proceeds over an acute illness phase as well as during recovery, while foetal monitoring is by comparison relatively brief. These disclaimers aside, a discussion of the psychological ramifications of such procedures would be incomplete without acknowledging the considerable controversy surrounding their use and the growing movement towards a return to natural childbirth methods. For example, a great deal has been written about the enjoyment of delivery, so that many women feel guilty or cheated if they have not enjoyed the moment of childbirth. Critics of the traditional medical delivery experience have asked what would be a comparable experience to labour under these conditions for a man, in order to alert the male medical profession to the problems of current obstetric practice. Some have suggested attaching a man to an intravenous drip, as women are commonly attached nowadays, and immobilizing his arm on his wedding night, and telling him to lie back and enjoy himself!

## Conclusion

Many advances have been made in the safety and accuracy of foetal diagnostic techniques. These introduce a further area of choice for the pregnant woman. Following her decision whether to proceed with or terminate the pregnancy, having decided to proceed, she may then discover the likelihood of the foetus being damaged and be able to elect a therapeutic termination. Such choices raise many ethical, moral and religious questions. Antenatal diagnosis is not acceptable to all, and cautionary statements have been made concerning the degree to which termination may follow relatively minor sources of dissatisfaction with the foetus, such as preferring not to have a child of that sex. A full discussion of these important issues is beyond the scope of this chapter. What is evident from the literature reviewed is that many eligible women are failing to take advantage of genetic counselling services. There is a need for education in this area, so that women have access to the information necessary to reach an informed decision.

Other procedures considered in this chapter, ultrasound and foetal monitoring, are also controversial, since it is often claimed they may serve staff needs more than the woman's. Research on this subject has shown ultrasound to be a generally acceptable and

## Antenatal foetal diagnosis 69

largely emotionally rewarding experience, particularly where specific verbal and visual feedback is made available to the woman. By including the partner in the examination, it may be possible to increase his emotional involvement in the pregnancy. As a result, the woman may receive more emotional and practical support during her pregnancy, both of which, as was seen in Chapter 2, assist in attenuating the impact of stress at this time. However, a discussion of this subject would not be complete without addressing the issue of safety, since many women are understandably anxious as to whether their foetus will be harmed by the ultrasound. Medical evidence on this point is reassuring. However, Towers (1981) draws an analogy with the apparent safety of X-rays, as used in the 1940s, before these were discovered to have harmful effects. It is clear from this that complacency on this point would be inappropriate and that further work is needed.

The practice of routinely attaching the foetus to monitoring equipment during labour remains controversial. To what extent does such a practice enhance safety and at what emotional cost to women? One problem with monitoring may be practical and attitudinal, in that the woman may feel cheated or neglected as staff focus their attention on the recording devices. It is important to ensure that, in parallel with monitoring, a woman's interpersonal and emotional needs are also met for, as will be seen in the following chapter, psychological state during labour will influence the pain experienced at this time.

Chapter 6

# The pain of labour

## Introduction

The changes that have taken place in the way in which childbirth is managed have had a major impact upon women's experience of labour and delivery. Childbirth has evolved from being a predominantly natural function to one controlled by the medical profession. Until the mid-twentieth century most births occurred at home. Within the comfort and familiarity of these surroundings, the pattern was one of high rates of infant mortality, maternal death and ill-health, partly as a result of what would be considered to be, by modern comparisons, substandard obstetric care. Although this picture no longer need apply to home deliveries, birth has become very much a medically controlled event, making it much safer for both mother and baby. With hospital deliveries now the norm, women typically find themselves delivering in the presence of strangers, in an unfamiliar setting, and as a result have been forced into a progressively more passive role. In spite of these changes, or some would argue as a result of them, the control of pain remains a prominent concern, so that while some women look forward to labour and delivery with a sense of completion and discovery, others express fears of being physically

# The pain of labour 71

damaged and view it as a personal assault (Schereshefsky and Yarrow 1973).

As mortality rates decline, so greater attention is given to providing effective means of pain control. Both chemical and psychological methods are widely used. Pain may remain the dominant memory of the experience for many women, and certainly fear of experiencing intolerable pain is one of the most commonly expressed concerns in antenatal clinics, as term approaches. Norr *et al.* (1977) suggested that women focus on two distinct dimensions of experience – pain and enjoyment – in describing childbirth. In their survey of 247 women, some women experienced little or no enjoyment, while others found giving birth to be one of the most joyful events of their lives. Pain and enjoyment were negatively correlated, with pain related to delivery anaesthesia, absence of pain control techniques and failure to utilize Lamaze preparation (Lamaze 1958). High levels of pain tended to interfere with enjoyment, although a significant proportion experienced both high enjoyment and high pain. Women with low levels of pain did not necessarily report high levels of enjoyment. Difficulty of delivery emerged as the only obstetric factor which had a direct effect on enjoyment. Methods of pain relief were important, although psychological factors also influenced enjoyment. The authors concluded that use of regional or general anaesthesia for difficult deliveries may have reduced the woman's ability to be sensitive, both to the enjoyable sensations of her own body and to social support from others in the delivery room; once again this emphasizes the importance of participation by the woman in the delivery experience.

## The nature of pain

The focus in this chapter will be on the pain associated with labour and delivery. Factors influencing this, both obstetric and psychological, will be examined, as well as the efficacy of psychological means of pain reduction in the form of birth preparation classes and psychoprophylaxis. In order to appreciate the context in which this work has been conducted it is necessary to draw upon what is known about the nature of pain, since evidence shows it to be influenced by a multitude of extrinsic and intrinsic stimuli. In addition to sensory input, cultural background, past experience, the meaning of the situation, personality, attention, arousal level and the prevailing reinforcement contingencies will all be involved in varying degrees. A model of pain which holds a simple, linear relationship between the amount of sensory input and the level of pain experienced is unable to account for the variation that exists. Psychological processes can be thought of as a flexible lens magnifying or reducing the amount of sensation that is felt. Those relevant to an understanding of childbirth pain will be considered, prior to an evaluation of the efficacy of pain reduction techniques.

The model depicted in Fig. 6 illustrates the range of concordance possible between the various levels of the pain experience. Four levels are distinguished: sensory input, conscious sensation, suffering and the behaviour brought about by a combination of sensation and suffering. The suffering component refers to the motivational aspect of pain; it is immediately aversive and prompts action to seek relief. While in many cases, particularly with acute pain, these components will reflect an internally consistent pattern, in that each will be activated by the former, on occasions desynchrony will be found. Thus, sensory input may be quiescent but pain behaviour in evidence. This may occur in chronic pain where pain behaviour may be maintained by prevailing reinforcement contigencies. For present purposes, the model offers a means of understanding the different levels at which the psychological pro-

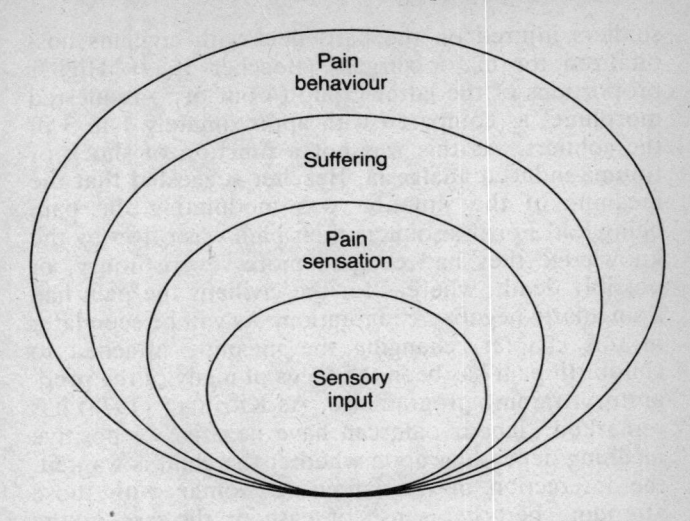

*Fig. 6* A model to illustrate the interplay between pain sensation and experience

cesses, to be described, may operate. They may change the pain threshold, and so influence whether or not sensory input is labelled as pain sensation rather than as pressure; they may determine the degree to which sensations have an aversive quality and they may affect the nature of pain behaviour produced, so that while some may display a stoical response, others may be more forthcoming in sharing their experience with those around them.

## Meaning of the situation

One of the first to draw explicit attention to the influence of the context in which pain occurs was American anaesthetist H. K. Beecher in the course of his classic studies of analgesic requirements. He compared US soldiers injured on the battlefield with civilians hospitalized for major surgery (Beecher 1959). Higher proportions of the latter group (4 out of 5) requested morphine, as compared with approximately 1 in 3 of the soldiers. As this was not a function of shock or trauma-induced analgesia, Beecher suggested that the meaning of the situation was modulating the pain being felt. For the soldiers their pain was offset by the knowledge they had escaped more severe injury, or possibly death, whereas for the civilians the pain had a singularly negative connotation. As will be seen later in this chapter, changing the meaning attached to childbirth pain has been the focus of many of the preparatory training programmes. As Kitzinger (1978) has remarked, 'labour pain can have negative or positive meaning depending upon whether the child is wanted, the interaction of the labouring woman with those attending her, her sense of ease or dis-ease in the environment provided for birth, her relationship with the father of the child and her attitude to her body throughout the reproductive process'.

## Is childbirth painful?

Proponents of natural childbirth, most notably Dick-Read (1944), have claimed that childbirth is not an inherently painful process but becomes so through the ambience in which it occurs. This perspective ascribes pain to secondary physiological processes produced by fear, and as a product of social, cultural and emotional influences. Such a viewpoint assumes pain to be a feature of Western societies and its proponents buttress these claims by drawing upon reports of childbirth in preliterate socities in which delivery is accomplished in the apparent absence of pain.

In order to appraise the influence of the meaning of the situation of childbirth, it is first necessary to consider the claim that pain is a product of Western birth practices. One of the most striking examples of childbirth without pain comes from reports of societies which practise couvade, in which the woman shows virtually no distress. In extreme cases she may continue to work in the field, tending her crop, until the birth becomes imminent, at which time, in tandem with her going into labour and delivering the baby, apparently without pain, her husband may take to bed and groan as though he were experiencing severe pain as *she* bears the child. Following the delivery, the man may remain in bed for several days in order to recover from his ordeal, while the woman returns to work in the fields.

While such reports abound, with respect to both childbirth and the endurance of noxious stimuli in the pursuit of societal rituals (Kosambi 1967), systematic appraisals of the evidence suggest that samples may not have been representative and the conclusions reached overgeneralized. Ford (1945) studied the problems of reproduction in sixty-four primitive societies and concluded, 'the popular impression of childbirth in primitive society as painless and easy is definitely contra-indicated by our cases. As a matter of fact, it is often prolonged and painful.' Moreover, parturition in animals clearly involves pain (Bonica 1967).

These reports can be reconciled with the views of physiologists that women have suffered pain in childbirth for as long as humans have existed on earth, by returning to the distinction made earlier between the experience and the expression of pain. It is the latter which is shaped and influenced by cultural and social-learning factors. It is a well established part of our culture for young girls to fear childbirth as they mature, an expectation which is difficult to dispel at the time of pregnancy. In the couvade situation we find no indication of pain behaviour in the woman, in spite of what may be substantial sensory input; whereas in the man, pain behaviour and suffering are evident, even though nociceptive input may be assumed to be absent. It can be concluded that while 'emotional, cultural and other factors can influence overt responses to pain, it is a normal consequence of the physiological processes of parturition' (Bonica 1975).

## Attitudes towards the delivery

The meaning attached to childbirth may influence pain levels both directly and indirectly. Indirectly, the effects may be mediated by raising anxiety levels or focusing attention on the pain experience. Directly, influences may arise through the way in which delivery has attained a surgical context, arousing all the negative emotions commonly associated with such a setting. The report of delivery pain has been analyzed in relation to attitudes towards the pregnancy expressed during the first trimester (Netterbladt *et al.* 1976). In a study of 78 primiparae, those reporting painful deliveries were more often consciously negative towards their pregnancy, more likely to have used insecure contraceptive techniques (suggesting conception may have been accidental), were more anxious about their deliveries and expressed greater ambivalence towards the prospect of motherhood. The authors conclude by stating, 'when childbirth implied more or less negative consequences for the woman, one of her ways of reacting was by reporting intense childbirth pain' (p. 220).

## Fear of pain

Of particular importance in the hospital setting is the influence of anxiety on pain thresholds and tolerance level. Pain threshold is reduced in the presence of elevated anxiety (Hill *et al.* 1952) and anxiety contributes to the aversiveness of the pain experience

(Melzack 1973). Labour and delivery are commonly anxiety-provoking situations, particularly for women in their first confinement. The fear of pain or anticipation of high pain levels will increase anxiety, which in turn will prove a self-fulfilling prophecy, because an increase in anxiety will lead to an increase in pain sensitivity (Melzack *et al.* 1963). Once again, childbirth preparation classes have attempted to provide information intended to reduce anticipatory anxiety, as well as teaching techniques of anxiety reduction to be utilized at the time on the assumption that one effect of increased maternal anxiety is heightened pain perception during labour. Klusman (1975) studied the effects of such information on anxiety by providing group instruction in the last trimester. Both ratings of 'fears for self' and 'fear for baby' were reduced by information, irrespective of its precise content. A significant association emerged between anxiety and pain ratings during the transition stage of labour (the hour before moving to the delivery room). Unfortunately, the failure to include a control group makes it impossible to exclude the effects of time alone in resolving anxiety levels.

## Personality

A further factor, worthy of special note, is the personality characteristics of those experiencing the pain. Experimental studies have consistently shown that introverts are more sensitive to pain stimuli and that those scoring higher on neuroticism display lower tolerance (Bond 1971). Clinical research has shown that whereas introverts may display greater sensitivity, extroverts complain more vociferously at a lower level of pain (Bond *et al.* 1976). Similar conclusions have emerged from studies of women during labour. Eysenck (1961), reporting personality data on a sample of 100 primiparae, found an association between extraversion and the likelihood of describing the pain as unbearable, thus confirming the reported tendency for extraverts to behaviourally exaggerate the painfulness of the situation, while introverts minimize it.

The relationship between personality, anxiety and pain during labour was investigated in a study of 80 women (Connolly *et al.* 1978). The sample was divided according to personality profiles measured on a standardized personality test (MMPI), and pain and anxiety measures were compared. Pain and anxiety levels rose over the course of labour, as might have been expected. Pain and anxiety were similar for normal and hysterical MMPI groups but different from those emerging as schizoid and anxious-depressive on the MMPI, with the latter groups displaying higher levels of pain and anxiety. The authors suggested that pain was secondary to anxiety, and that this was affected by personality differences in preferred coping style. The lower scores of the hysterical group reflected their predisposition to utilize denial and conversion coping strategies, thereby becoming less consciously aware of their anxiety state than schizoid and anxious-depressive personality types.

To summarize the evidence on personality, it appears this may have a direct effect on sensory processing by modulating arousal levels and trait anxiety. It may influence the way in which the pain is manifested, which may in turn influence staff behaviour in terms of the administration of medication. In addition to its influence on the predisposition to become anxious, personality may be related to the coping style habitually adopted in the face of stress. The adequacy of the coping strategy will depend on the precise nature of the circumstances. There are indications to suggest that those who attempt to exercise control, whether cognitive (such as distraction) or behavioural (such as avoidance or, failing that, relaxation), may cope better than those adopting a passive, helpless response.

## Drug needs

Before going on to focus on childbirth pain, it is necessary to introduce one further factor – not directly affecting the pain experience itself, but none the less entering into the picture in the clinical setting. It would be a mistake to assume that patients who experience pain receive medication titrated to their pain needs by the attending clinical staff. The environment in which the pain is being experienced exercises a powerful influence on the drugs received. In particular, the perceptions, preferences and stereotypes held by the medical staff will affect the dispensing of pain relief medication. Bond and Pilowsky (1966) showed nursing attitudes on an oncology ward to be more closely related to drug administration than to patients' subjective reports of pain. Similarly, Keats (1956) showed that patients on public wards received less medication than those on private wards. In the obstetric context, the obstetrician's personal stereotypes and appraisal of the woman's need for medication may influence what she receives. Similarly, requests for epidural anaesthesia may be a function of their availability and the way in which women are introduced to this option.

## The management of childbirth pain

Strange as it may now seem, attempts to ease the pain of childbirth have met with opposition in the past, predominantly from religious groups. Upon the introduction of anaesthesia in the middle of the eighteenth century, members of the Catholic Church (who were exclusively male), objected because the Bible was interpreted as advocating pain in childbirth as punishment for 'eating the forbidden fruit'. As the Lord told Eve in the Book of Genesis, 'I will greatly multiply thy sorrow and thy conception; in sorrow thou shalt bring forth children.' However, criticism abated, from the Anglician Church at least, when Queen Victoria consented to the use of chloroform while giving birth to her seventh child.

Having sanctioned the use of pain control methods, we now find chemical methods in almost universal use. It should be acknowledged that opposition from the Catholic Church continued, as it was only in the 1950s that a papal decree accepted painless childbirth as consistent with the teachings of the Catholic Church. Opposition has not been confined to the Church, however, as none other than Helen Deutsch, a distinguished psychoanalyst, remarked as recently as 1942 that pain in childbirth was essential for the process of mother-infant bonding! Among the factors influencing bonding which will be developed in detail in the following chapter, the experience of pain does not emerge as facilitative.

## The mechanics of childbirth pain

In order to evaluate methods of pain relief, it is necessary to have some understanding of the mechanisms of pain at this time. Although the precise neurophysiological and biochemical mechanisms producing pain during the various stages of labour and vaginal delivery have not been conclusively determined, data suggest it is due to (a) dilatation of the cervix; (b) contraction and distension of the uterus; (c) distention of the outlet, vulva and perineum; and (d) a number of other mechanisms, including traction and pressure on the adnexa and parietal peritoneum; pressure on and stretching of the bladder, rectum and other pain-sensitive structures in the pelvis; pressure on one or more roots of the lumbosacral plexus, and reflex skeletal muscle spasm; and vasospasm in those structures supplied by the same spinal cord segments that supply the uterus.

Physical factors that influence labour pain include:

(a) the intensity and duration of uterine contractions; (b) the degree to which the cervix dilates and how rapidly this occurs; (c) distension of the perineal tissue; (d) age, parity, the condition of the cervix at the outset of labour, the size of the foetus in relation to the birth canal and the patient's general health. Fatigue, loss of sleep, anaemia, general debility and malnutrition exert an influence on the patient's tolerance of the experience. In general, elderly primiparae experience longer and more painful labours than their younger counterparts. The cervix of a multipara begins to soften even before the onset of labour and is less sensitive than that of a primipara. The intensity of uterine contractions in early labour tends to be higher in primiparae than in multiparae, whereas in the later stages of labour the opposite becomes the case.

As was mentioned earlier, pain in labour has many potentially debilitating effects, hence the emphasis on reduction. The physiological effects are intertwined with the alterations produced by the process of labour, in addition to the effects of psychological state. Pain during labour may increase cardiac output by between 15 to 60 per cent, as well as increasing blood pressure and cardiac rate. In some instances severe pain may produce disturbances of cardiac rhythm and changes in the T-wave of the electrocardiogram, decrease in coronary blood flow and pressure changes in the cardiac chambers. It may also produce severe hyperventilation with consequent decrease in cerebral and uterine blood flow, with attendant hazards for the foetus. Other effects include alterations in the functioning of the uterus, gastrointestinal tract, kidney and urinary bladder and reflex spasm of skeletal muscles, as well as the possibility of precipitating nausea and vomiting.

## Pharmacological pain control

Surveys of obstetric records show that only a minority

of women decline medication altogether in controlling their pain. We carried out two separate surveys of consecutive series of primiparae at King's College Hospital and found, out of total sample sizes of 129 and 101, the number undergoing totally 'unassisted' deliveries to be 5 in each case (Campbell *et al.* 1982; Reading *et al.* 1982b). Drugs most commonly prescribed for vaginal delivery are pethidine, inhalation analgesia (Entonox) and regional anaesthesia (epidural). The British Births Survey (Chamberlain *et al.* 1975) revealed that nearly 70 per cent of women received pethidine during labour. Inhalation analgesia is rarely effective in isolation, owing to its short duration of effect, requiring precise matching of inhalations to contractions. Many units are now able to offer epidural blocks on demand. Where this is accomplished, pain relief is reported to be high, with 60 per cent experiencing total relief and 20 to 30 per cent reasonable reduction of the pain. Other pharmacological interventions include the administration of minor tranquillizers and paracervical and pudendal nerve blocks.

As is the case with many medical treatments, the benefit needs to be balanced against the cost, in this case primarily that to the foetus. As has been seen, uncontrolled levels of pain may endanger the foetus by causing hyperventilation resulting in foetal anoxia. Pethidine may have the disadvantage of causing excessive drowsiness which may interfere with the woman's perception and emotional reaction towards the neonate. Also, the pain relief it provides may be poor for a proportion of women and it is not possible to identify such mothers in advance (Rosen 1977). Irrespective of its effect on the mother, it is well established that pethidine crosses the placenta, diminishes respiratory adaptation at birth, and may lower the Apgar score (this refers to a means of grading newborns, with 0, 1 or 2 points awarded for each of five signs: heart rate, respiratory effort, muscle tone, reflex irritability and colour) by one or two points (Chamberlain *et al.* 1975). Although this may be of little significance to the full-term baby, it may present more of a problem in the case of a premature delivery. Studies examining longer-term effects have identified an association with depressed feeding patterns (Dubignon *et al.* 1969) and lowered scores on a number of neurobehavioural measures (Brackbill *et al.* 1974).

Few adverse effects of epidural blocks on foetal and neonatal wellbeing have been reported, with the exception of a reduction in muscle tone (Scanlon 1976), which may affect feeding. There are indications, however, that the increasing use of epidural anaesthesia may affect the delivery, since the resultant loss of reflex stimulation from the perineum diminishes muscle power and the woman's urge to push. This has led to an increased need for forceps, explaining the increased incidence of episiotomies and lacerations (Alberman 1977).

## Psychological methods of pain control

The inevitable drawbacks of pharmacological methods of pain reduction reinforce the need to develop alternatives. The rationale for implementing psychological methods can be drawn from two sources: (a) the evidence reviewed earlier demonstrating the influence of psychological state on pain: (b) the success of psychological methods in relieving pain control in other settings (e.g., Barber and Adrian-Barber 1982). Surprisingly, it has not only been chemical means of ameliorating pain which have been criticized and subjected to prolonged controversy – psychoprophylactic techniques have been also criticized for interfering with a natural process. In spite of this, extensive use has been made of psychological methods, dating back to the last century (Bonwill 1880). In fact they may be regarded as precursors of the current application of such approaches in the full range of pain conditions, particularly chronic pain.

Before considering evidence on efficacy, we will consider the historical roots of psychoprophylactic techniques: Dick-Read's (1944) natural childbirth; Velvovsky et al.'s (1960) 'Pavlovian' methods; and Lamaze (1958). The latter derived from Fernard Lamaze's contact with Russian methods which he introduced to the West, bearing his own name. All contain common ingredients in the form of information, breathing instructions and relaxation exercises. In fact the similarity between the techniques led to acrimonious debate among their proponents, as Wessel and Ellis accused the Russians of rediscovering the wheel in claiming their technique to be new (see Dick-Read 1972). Irrespective of their origins, in combination these movements have attained current wide-scale availability.

As Beck and Hall (1978) point out in their review of the evidence, irrespective of the particular methods currently advocated, at least three common ingredients can be identified. The first consists of providing accurate information about the processes of labour and delivery. Experimental work has documented the efficacy of information in reducing pain sensation (Johnson 1973), although clinical trials have been less consistent (Reading 1979). It appears that information needs to be combined with advice on how to cope with the impending sensations (Langer et al. 1975). The second and third ingredients satisfy this object by focusing on relaxation exercises and breathing control respectively. The means by which muscle relaxation can be achieved have varied from the use of progressive muscle relaxation (Jacobson 1939), cognitive relaxation (Rybstein-Blinchik 1979), to the use of hypnosis (Barber 1977). A fourth factor, more recently acknowledged, concerns the involvement of the partner both in the birth and in assisting the woman to utilize her training in relaxation and breathing. This remains perhaps the most controversial element, which is unfortunate, because evidence suggests that the active involvement of the partner may offer a potent means of pain control. Kitzinger (1980) has offered some pertinent observations on the status of the partner in the delivery room. She depicts a scene in which the amount of sterile clothing adorning those present at the birth is inversely proportional to status, with the consultant merely wearing surgical mask and the woman's partner swathed from head to toe. Moreover, the man may be made to feel superfluous and ordered from the room at the first sign of difficulty. Also, not all women feel comfortable with their partner in attendance. As with all coping strategies this one needs to be adapted to the patient's individual needs. However, where the partner is able to make a positive contribution, the effects on pain appear to be substantial (Cogan *et al*. 1976).

Evidence on the efficacy of preparation on pain is mixed and difficult to interpret owing to the inconsistent methodology employed. In considering this issue it is illuminating to understand the context in which these techniques have gained acceptance. Obstetricians have become aware of potentially adverse effects of chemical anaesthesia and analgesia on the foetus. Parallel to professional considerations, the influence of the growing lay movement, increasingly concerned with the adverse effects of the medicalization of the obstetric service, should be recognized. By comparison, psychological methods incur no risk to the mother or foetus, may allay ante-natal anxiety by providing goal-oriented tasks, and have the potential of facilitating delivery.

## Who uses psychological methods?

Not all women take advantage of birth preparation classes. As was seen in Chapter 3, the level of adherence to health advice varies considerably. The question of who takes advantage of such classes has been studied. Cave (1978) compared the demographic characteristics of users and non-users in New York. Significant differences in social characteristics were found, with users more likely to be of higher social class, higher income, older, more educated, with better-educated partners and higher occupations than non-users. Such results conform to the pattern reported in the utilization of other preventive health measures, such as vaccines, detection kits or cervical testing programmes. The characteristics of the non-users are reminiscent of those identified in Chapter 3 as displaying low take-up of antenatal services in general.

## Conclusions

A number of general conclusions can be drawn. That childbirth can be painful and that pain is a principal concern of women prior to delivery is beyond dispute. It is also well established that a number of psychological processes exert an important modulating influence on the pain experience. While pharmacological approaches may provide effective pain control for the majority of women, two provisos are indicated. First, pain control may be at a cost, in terms of maternal awareness, sensitivity and control, as well as possible adverse effects on the foetus. Second, these methods will not be uniformly effective. Although drugs may affect the foetus, these risks need to be balanced against those to the foetus in the absence of pain control. In this context – that of the prominence of pain and the problems with drugs – it is evident that non-pharmacological means of improving the comfort of the woman in labour by the use of psychological methods of pain control are important. These may focus on the pain directly, through teaching distraction or other pain control techniques, or attempt to alter pain indirectly, by reducing anxiety levels. Rather than debate the merits of one approach versus the other, it may be that psychological approaches can be used to potentiate the action of drugs and so, where these are used, ensure that dosage is kept to a minimum. This will not be the last discussion of pain. It will be returned to in the final chapter, owing to its continuing prominence in the postpartum period.

Chapter 7

# Bonding: reactions to the neonate

The emphasis of the previous chapter was on the woman's experience during delivery and attempts to reduce her pain and 'suffering'. This chapter will be concerned with her reactions to the neonate and the subsequent interaction during the first few days postpartum. In recent years, considerable attention has been given to the provision of conditions at birth conducive to mother-baby bonding. In fact, the notion of bonding, in one form or another, permeates much current obstetric and midwifery practice and teaching. Emphasis is being laid on providing the mother with the opportunity for extended contact with her neonate, with many obstetric units routinely offering immediate skin-to-skin contact in their efforts to enhance the 'bond'. The concept of bonding and the influence of obstetric practice will be considered in the first part of this chapter, followed by examination of the factors influencing the mother's psychological state over the first few days postpartum.

## Bonding

With the writings of Klaus and Kennell (1976) the notion of bonding has assumed a prominent place in the paediatrician's vocabulary. Although the practice of nursery care, in which the mother is separated from her baby for prolonged periods, has largely disappeared (with the exception of babies requiring intensive neonatal care), the authors draw attention to other factors which are believed to facilitate the bonding process. These include ambulatory labour, reducing lighting and noise in the delivery room, excluding non-essential or observing staff members, involving the woman's partner, dispensing with stirrups, a more upright posture for delivery and a conservative attitude towards episiotomy. More extreme examples of this trend can be found in the advocacy of Leboyer deliveries in which, in an attempt to lessen the trauma of birth, the newborn is bathed in order to minimize the transition from the mother's womb (Leboyer 1975). Although there is little compelling evidence in support of Leboyer (Nelson *et al.* 1980), the importance attached to mother-baby bonding is illustrated by the fact that recently issued (1979) guidelines by the American Medical Association stipulated the conditions necessary for the promotion of attachment and bonding of mothers to infants.

## The consequences of 'failure to bond'

Parallel to changes in clinical practice, research has attempted to document the consequences of bonding failures. This research has had two main elements: (a) an evaluation of the effects of certain aspects of obstetric practice (such as separating mother and baby); and (b) investigations of the potential benefit of providing conditions at birth (such as immediate skin-to-skin contact) intended to facilitate the bonding process. As was seen in Chapter 4, the focus on the postpartum period has tended to obscure the importance of the antenatal period in facilitating the development of maternal feelings. Experiences during pregnancy will influence the degree to which the woman is adequately prepared for the delivery experience and the role of motherhood. Before examining the evidence, a number of conceptual issues will be addressed.

## Critical periods?

The term 'bonding' has been used with varying connotations and to denote a variety of processes. It has been implicated in as diverse health problems as hyperemesis in pregnancy, failure of the baby to thrive and child abuse some years following the birth. A basic distinction has been drawn between the concepts of bonding and attachment, since researchers have tended to use these terms interchangeably (Campbell and Taylor 1979). The former may be characterized as primarily unidirectional, occurring rapidly and facilitated by physical contact. Attachment may be considered a gradual process, dependent upon reciprocal interaction between mother and infant and facilitated by predominantly psychological processes. It is the former which will be considered here.

The origins of the concept derive from animal ethologists' observations that particular species-specific behaviour patterns are highly predictable and are consistently elicited by certain stimulus configurations, especially when the organism is in a state of biological readiness. Analogous processes are believed to operate in humans. For example, Klaus and Kennell (1976) suggest the existence of a sensitive period following the delivery during which the mother is most likely to develop strong affectional ties to her infant. As a corollary, they suggest that separation at this time is believed to have adverse effects on mothering which may persist for some months, thereby increasing the likelihood of subsequent child abuse. This viewpoint has its antecedents in psychoanalytic theory (Winnicott 1958), which places importance on the immediate postpartum period and attaches particular emphasis to permitting unhindered physical contact at this time.

## The adverse effects of separation

Owing to the ethical problems of conducting research in humans on this topic, studies evaluating the damaging effects of mother-neonate separation have had to rely upon retrospective data on the epidemiology of parenting failures. The data indicate that a high proportion of premature and sick infants are abused or fail to thrive. For example, Lynch and Roberts (1977) examined the birth records of 50 children who had been abused and found that 21 of them had been admitted to intensive care units following delivery, compared with only 5 from a control group of non-abused children. A failure of the mothers to form an adequate bond after delivery was invoked as an explanation of subsequent abuse, in spite of the absence of a direct assessment of bonding failure. Similarly, O'Connor *et al.* (1977) reported rooming-in (keeping mother and infant together) to be associated with a decreased incidence of parenting failure. Only one case of child abuse was reported for the mothers who roomed-in, as compared with nine cases of battering, neglect, or failure to thrive among the 158 infants given traditional nursery care. It should be noted that rooming mothers were not provided with increased early contact, but were united with their babies several hours after the delivery.

Research of this kind encounters a number of problems in attempting to disentangle causal processes. It is seldom possible to control for the many other variables affecting outcome, such as poverty, family disorganization, parental psychopathology and poor antenatal care, all of which are associated with a higher incidence of premature and high-risk babies, as well as distortions in parenting. Studies often fail to assess the outcome of the entire population admitted to intensive care units, rather than the proportion subsequently abused. Direct evidence of impaired interaction is rarely available, for if separation due to neonatal ill health results in an impairment of the bonding process, this might be reflected in the observed interaction patterns. Studies addressing this question have not shown unequivocally less affectionate or appropriate mothering among mothers of sick infants (Leifer *et al.* 1972).

It can be concluded that there is no direct evidence implicating bonding problems resulting from obstetric outcome in later abuse and neglect. The causes of the latter are clearly multiple and complex. Egeland and Vaughn (1981) draw attention to the relevance of certain personality characteristics of the mother, present before the birth, which may affect both her capacity to become bonded to her baby and her subsequent mothering. Such women may be less diligent in seeking antenatal care and as a result have more premature and otherwise vulnerable infants. In this case, failure to form a bond would be a manifestation of a more pervasive problem and not necessarily the cause of later mothering disorders.

## The benefits of early contact

The benefits of enhancing early contact have been studied in relation to breast-feeding patterns and early interaction processes. An association has emerged between early skin-to-skin contact and suckling within the first hour after birth. In a study carried out in Guatemala, the effects of extra early contact on mother-infant interaction were assessed at twelve hours, one month and one year (Klaus *et al.* 1972). The extra contact group, consisting of 16 primigravidae, were provided with their naked infants for one hour during the first 3 hours after birth, and for 5 hours each day for the next 3 days. A control group received routine care, consisting of brief contact at delivery, after 12 hours and thereafter at four-hourly feeds. The assessments at 72 hours indicated more pronounced attachment behaviour among the extra contact group. Data collected at one month and one year (Kennell *et al* 1974) showed mothers in this group to display more affectionate and positive attitudes towards their infants than the controls. Although the intention was to evaluate the importance of a critical period following delivery, it is evident that the women in the two conditions differed substantially in access to the baby over the first four days postpartum.

Dechateau (1979) studied the effects of additional physical contact at three months and one year. In this study, the experimental manipulation consisted of providing women with 25 minutes of skin-to-skin contact with the baby, commencing within 20 minutes of delivery. A matched group of twenty controls were denied this initial contact but subsequently received identical care. More pronounced attachment behaviour was evident at both 3 and 12 months for the additional-contact mothers compared with the control group. Further analyses revealed these differences to be derived from mother-boy interactions, whereas interactions between mothers and female infants in the two experimental conditions were comparable. The women themselves could not be distinguished on psychological assessment, although babies in the early contact group were more responsive at three months. This disparity raises the possibility that the extra contact group may have contained a higher proportion of babies who were more alert and positive in mood from the outset.

Once again, the dependent variables studied in this context are multi-determined and not necessarily an index of bonding. Thus, breast-feeding has been used as an index of bonding in a number of studies, although, as will be seen, it is clear that a host of other factors will influence both the decision to breastfeed and its duration. Insufficient attention has been given to the neonate's capacity to influence the interaction process. For example, premature and sick infants may be more difficult to care for, regardless of the skill of the caretaker. It has been established that individual differences exist from birth in the infant's ability to elicit interaction and in such behaviour as crying, cuddliness and visual alertness (Korner 1971). Observations of early feeding have shown that more alert and responsive infants elicit more stimulation (Condon and Sandler 1979). The infant's role is most dramatically seen in the case of prematurity, as the pre-term infant's frail appearance and lack of responsiveness may be a factor in delaying attachment, owing to the absence of reciprocity. This is based on the view that the baby's characteristics in terms of appearance and responsiveness play a large part in releasing attachment and care-giving behaviour in the mother (Jeffcoate *et al.* 1979).

## Subjective reactions of the woman to her baby

In addition to behavioural observations, studies have examined women's subjective reactions upon first seeing and holding their baby. It appears that considerable variation exists, with a proportion reporting predominantly negative or detached emotional reactions towards the neonate. Newton and Newton (1962) studied the initial reactions of 692 women and found 31 per cent to be pleased, 13 per cent indifferent and 1 per cent disgusted. Robson and Kumar (1980) asked 119 primiparae, seven days after delivery, to comment upon their initial reactions. Of the sample, 40 per cent were recorded as displaying initial indifference, while 13 per cent had mixed feelings towards the neonate. These negative feelings dissipated rapidly and were unrelated to postpartum depression, breast-feeding or subsequent emotional outbursts against the child.

The failure of mothers to display uniformly positive feelings has been considered a normal variant, or as conferring an advantage in that bonding may be deferred until the baby's survival is assured (MacFarlane 1974). Robson and Kumar (1980) reported an association between receiving an amniotomy (articifial rupturing of the membranes), maternal indifference and pain, as indexed by subjective report and administration of high doses of pethidine. Newton and Newton (1962) concluded that those women who appeared less disturbed during labour and remained calm and co-operative throughout the delivery were more likely to accept their babies upon first seeing them. These findings introduce the possibility that maternal reactions may be a function of the level of stress experienced during labour and delivery.

It is helpful to draw upon research which has examined reactions to stressful medical procedures, in order to appreciate the way in which stress at this time may interfere with the release of maternal feelings. Stress is a function of subjective perceptions, with wide individual variation in the degree to which ostensibly identical circumstances will be appraised as stressful (Lazarus 1975). Similarly, the preferred way of coping in response to stress will vary, with a proportion of patients predisposed to adopt an avoidant coping style (Cohen and Lazarus 1973). Such a perspective provides a framework within which a detached or negative emotional state at the time of delivery may be viewed as an adaptive reaction elicited by the rigours of labour and delivery, rather than as the mother's perception of the neonate *per se*. This suggests that initial maternal indifference would be expected to dissipate rapidly, a proposition confirmed by the results of Robson and Kumar (1980).

## Fulfilling expectations

It is revealing to reflect upon the normative influences on maternal reactions to the neonate. Danziger (1979) suggests 'the rules for proper birthing conduct are laid down, rather than negotiated with individual patients'! These norms often have the appearance of satisfying the needs of staff routine rather than the woman's experience of contractions and assume that the woman will remain passive and compliant during labour. Attempts on her part to discuss the advisability of changes in obstetric procedure, or whether an episiotomy is desirable, may be met by staff declarations of their superior ability to judge. Similarly, calmness during birth and initial acceptance of the baby are the socially approved reactions. Patients failing to conform to normative expectations may be labelled deviant.

Such calm acceptance of the baby may not be a uniform response but be related, amongst other factors, to the stress experienced during the delivery. Socializing influences may constrain women to co-operate and to express delight upon first seeing their baby (Werts *et al.* 1965). Those whose emotional reactions fail to match their preconceived expectations may experience guilt and self-doubt about their feelings toward the baby. These might be diminished if attention were given to this issue in the course of preparation classes, where women could be warned of the possibility of a mixed reaction to the baby, and advised that negative feelings tend to dissipate rapidly over the first few days postpartum.

## Breast is best

In reviewing the evidence on the implications of bonding failures, breast-feeding emerged as a possible index of the adequacy of the bond. As was stated then, data on breast-feeding patterns needs to be interpreted cautiously, since many factors enter into both the decision to breast-feed, and for how long this is pursued. In general, studies show a disparity between the numbers stating their intention to breast-feed and those actually accomplishing this for any length of time. This may not be surprising when we take into consideration the context in which information on intentions is obtained. During pregnancy women will be asked their feeding preference – breast or bottle. This is recorded in the case notes, and possibly information as to the nutritional benefits of breast milk over formula milk will be given, where a preference for bottle feeding is elicited. However, this answer will be given in the context of the prevailing attitude among health professionals that breast is best. It may be assumed, therefore, that at least some of those answers elicited in pregnancy will be influenced by the woman's perception of this prevailing cultural norm.

The failure of many women to continue breast-feeding is receiving growing attention. Evidence on the merits of breast milk appears overwhelming. In addition to having the potential to facilitate the mother-neonate bond, there are the many physiological attractions of breast milk. The nutritional constitutents of breast milk provide the neonate with added resistance to the penetration of intestinal organisms, adequate vitamin needs and a reduction in the incidence of allergies, ulcerative colitis and infant sudden death syndrome. Maternal advantages go beyond enhancing bonding, since breast-feeding may diminish the likelihood of breast carcinoma and offer contraceptive cover during the postpartum period (Weinstein 1980). In order to understand the problem, it is necessary to appreciate both the attractions of breast-feeding and its particular disadvantages, from the woman's standpoint. Many obstacles are cited: the lack of facilities, dislike of the schedule, infections, embarrassment, fear as to the cosmetic effects, and so on. From a behavioural perspective, it would be necessary to establish the extent to which such factors would be responsive to educational efforts.

It is possible that the failure to devote anything more than brief attention to preference in the antenatal period and acceptance of the woman's preference at face value, where she states an intention to breast-feed, may represent a failure to take advantage of the opportunity to provide counselling at this stage. Similarly, the provision of information and education in the postpartum period may avoid unnecessary problems caused by misunderstandings, fear of failure, etc. Ultimately, however, many of the problems may be found to derive from the value placed upon the breast as a sexual attribute, particularly revered in Western cultures. To quote from Weinstein (1980):

> The breast has always been a glorified portion of the female anatomy, from early Greek sculpture through Renaissance art to our current day movies and magazines. The breast has been constrained by the tight corsets of the Victorian era, enlarged by the padding of twentieth century brassières, and allowed to assume a position of minimal or no support as current fashion dictates. Although most people will agree that this portion of the female anatomy is beautiful to behold, the modern-day woman is often not utilizing this appendage for its major function, that of newborn nutrition.

It may be necessary to acknowledge that the cultural tide of social and sexual pressure is a strong one, and to focus on changing male values and the broader cultural milieu, rather than continue to scapegoat women. The lack of concern with male participation in this aspect of care-giving, is a reflection of traditional values that men should be minimally involved. Thus, male reactions to their wives breast-feeding has been seldom considered (Waletzky 1979).

## Intrauterine and neonatal death

A consideration of bonding would be incomplete without reference to the impact of neonatal or intrauterine death. With the advances made in perinatal care and monitoring, and the establishment of neonatal care units, the chances of survival of low birthweight babies have increased considerably (Baum *et al.* 1977). In spite of this, statistical records indicate a foetal mortality rate of 11 per cent per 1,000 and neonatal also at this level. When death occurs the parents involved experience a grief reaction similar to that felt when older loved ones die. What data there are suggest little difference in the grief response to any type of perinatal death. Kennel *et al.* (1970) interviewed twenty women whose babies had died and assessed the presence of five indicators of grief: sadness, loss of appetite, inability to sleep, preoccupation and inability to return to normal activity. One finding was the lack of association between their derived 'mourning score' and the length of the baby's life. This is significant, since it calls into question earlier assumptions that grief at this time is dissimilar to that experienced at the loss of an adult. For example, Deutsch (1943) believed it reflected the nonfulfilment of wish fantasy.

The methodology developed by Kennell *et al.* (1970) was utilized in a retrospective survey of grief reactions to deaths in the perinatal period by Peppers and Knapp (1980). They expanded their grief indices by including difficulty in concentration, anger, guilt, failure to accept reality, time confusion, exhaustion, lack of strength, depression and repetitive dreams of the lost child. Women were required to rate themselves on each variable, yielding an overall grief index for the sixty-five women studied. The scores for women experiencing a miscarriage, stillbirth and neonatal death were comparable, with a less intense reaction reported by women who subsequently gave birth to a healthy child, and more intense reactions in women with a history of pregnancy difficulties.

The reactions of the father have not been studied, yet it is clear that he shares the grieving process, although he may feel obliged to conceal this in order to support his partner. The strain imposed on the relationship also needs to be acknowledged, particularly with respect to the rate at which the grief feelings are resolved. This may lead to problems through misunderstandings about the other partner's grief reactions. Similarly, existing children may share in these difficulties, either directly or by changes in their parents' behaviour towards them.

Caring for the parents in the event of perinatal death raises important considerations. In the case of a stillbirth the woman may find herself falling between specialists in that obstetricians may consider their role completed, while the paediatrician sees no reason to become involved. The available evidence attests to the depth of investment in the foetus which may develop over the course of the pregnancy, and the needs of women who experience a loss. The benefits of seeing the baby and being kept informed are known. Hospital obstetric units can be isolating, lonely places at the best of times, and such feelings will be magnified if the staff feel hesitant about contact. The woman with a dead or malformed baby may feel as if the staff are avoiding her, which may be the case, owing to their own discomfort and difficulties. As Sahu (1981) points out, the woman whose baby has died continues to have medical needs. Engorged breasts will be an additional painful reminder of the dead baby and sensitive care at this time is important.

## The father's role

Discussion of the bonding process would be incomplete without acknowledging the role of the father. Men have become much more active participants in the process of childbearing, accompanying women to antenatal clinic appointments, participating in birth preparation classes and attending the actual birth. Observational studies of neonatal interaction with both parents have revealed the father to be as nurturant and responsive as the mother to infant cues, such as vocalizations and mouth movements (Parke *et al.* 1979).

## Conclusions

A number of conclusions relating to mother-neonate bonding in the postpartum period are possible (Reading 1983): (a) that prematurity and separation at birth may be associated with subsequent parenting difficulties, although moderating variables, such as the pre-existing personality characteristics of the mother and other socio-demographic variables, need to be taken into consideration; (b) when parent bonds do break down, it may be more appropriate to look for multiple causes, rather than to identify one very early event as the predisposing trauma; (c) there is little doubt that any hospital procedure which makes the mother feel more comfortable or more competent to care for her baby will be a positive influence on the development of the bond, hence the potentially disruptive effects of separation; (d) as Rutter (1979) has indicated, 'the fact that fathers or adoptive parents develop close ties suggests that bonding may most readily occur at delivery, but it is evident that it may occur later'; (e) the belief in the primacy of the mother-neonate bond has tended to obscure the role of the father. Research on the father is particularly germane in view of the increasing tendency for the father to be present during the delivery. Greenberg and Morris (1976) found that those fathers who were present at the delivery displayed greater comfort holding the baby and believed themselves to be more able to recognize it than fathers whose first contact occurred when the baby was presented to them by the nursing staff; (f) the inclusion of the antenatal period in research evaluations will indicate the pattern of change during the pregnancy and the importance of this for subsequent mother-neonate bonding.

Chapter 8

# The postpartum and beyond

The intention of the present work has been to present a perspective on those psychological aspects of pregnancy that lend themselves to an empirical analysis. As a result, scant mention has been made of intrapsychic conflicts or motives; rather the focus has been on the effects of the pregnant woman's behaviour and on ways of inducing behaviour change. Such an orientation is consistent with the current emphasis on 'behavioural medicine', which gives explicit recognition to the importance of life-style factors in disease aetiology and the maintenance of health. As was seen in Chapter 3, a woman's behaviour during pregnancy may adversely affect foetal and neonatal health and development. Just as the pendulum in medicine has swung away from the germ model of disease to recognition of the importance of life style, so there are indications that within obstetrics we may be seeing greater balance between the use of high technology and ensuring that sufficient attention is given to psychological and behavioural factors, such as have been identified in the preceding chapters. For example, Kitzinger (1978) has remarked upon the need for a supportive and sensitive environment in order to reduce what she refers to as 'environmental stress' at this time. In a survey of British maternity hospitals, supportive and sensitive environments were discovered to be almost uniformly lacking.

This perspective may be further developed by suggesting that pregnancy may be an optimum time at which to introduce preventive health care considerations to the woman and other members of the family unit. Comment has already been made on the dual payoff of appropriate behaviour change during pregnancy. This refers to the reduction of risk to the foetus and, where this change endures, the long-term benefits to the woman's own health status in the months and years following the delivery. Thus, encouraging women to cease smoking while pregnant is a worthwhile aim in itself. Should this be successful and the woman continue to be a non-smoker, the benefits become manifold. Speculation has been made that pregnancy may be a time of increased receptivity to health education efforts, owing to the motivation to safeguard the health of the foetus. If this assumption is substantiated, there may be an opportunity to use the time of pregnancy to inculcate a broad range of adaptive health habits. Such a strategy becomes particularly attractive when the numbers involved are considered – it is an event which touches the majority of the population. The perspective may be further broadened by including the male role. Not only may the man provide his partner with beneficial support in her efforts to ensure the viability of the pregnancy, his involvement may also provide an opportunity to educate him in preventive health measures. There are few opportunities for contact with men, unlike women, through family planning and antenatal services, and so pregnancy may provide a largely untapped opportunity to attempt to facilitate appropriate health behaviour in the male.

### The unkindest cut of all

Consideration of pregnancy would be limited if no

mention were made of the postpartum period and beyond. The fear of experiencing a deep depression following the birth, the stress of caring for the baby and developing the necessary mothering skills are just a few of the concerns expressed by women during the weeks before delivery. One particular area of concern is the likelihood of having an episiotomy (the cut made in the vaginal wall to facilitate the passage of the baby's head) at the time of delivery and its effects on future sexual activity and enjoyment. There are indications to suggest that this procedure may have been over-utilized, since the incidence rates for first births vary across hospitals. It may be greater in teaching hospitals where staff have less experience and so prefer to take this precautionary measure rather than run the risk of allowing the woman to tear (which is uncontrolled and more difficult to repair). An episiotomy is associated with pain during the first few weeks postpartum; the level of pain and the likelihood of additional problems appears to be related to the way in which the cut is sutured. In many hospitals there is a wait for suturing to be performed. Follow-up studies indicate that a proportion of episiotomy sutures break down or become infected.

The relevance of this problem to a discussion of psychological aspects of pregnancy emerged from a survey carried out of women completing their first pregnancy and having an episiotomy (Reading *et al* 1982b). The absence of detailed information on the nature of the procedure and what to expect in the recovery period was striking. Some women assumed that a complication had emerged when the midwife told them she was going to have to give them a cut. Others failed to bring problems in the postpartum period to the attention of their doctor, because they believed the level of pain to be unavoidable. It appears that women could benefit from knowing which problems will subside in time and which warrant medical help. By seeking prompt care, secondary difficulties associated with sexual performance may be avoided. A further finding from the study was the inadequacy of the six-week postpartum appointment as a means of assessing sexual problems, since few women have become sexually active by this time. This question needs to be also asked at a later date.

## The march of technology

The complex moral, ethical and legal issues raised by the development of techniques of foetal diagnosis and visualization were alluded to in Chapter 5. These techniques may both increase and reduce the woman's right to decide the fate of her foetus. The practice of selective abortion of the malformed foetus is a well-established facility in antenatal care. Those women who find such an option unacceptable need not undergo screening or diagnostic tests. But what of the situation where an abnormality is detected late in the pregnancy, possibly by ultrasound, and the woman and staff disagree over management, with the latter responding to the needs of the foetus? This refers to the circumstance where a woman, upon learning her foetus is badly damaged, prefers not to undergo heroic attempts to save it in the event of a complication occurring. Thus, she may decline the use of a foetal monitor in labour and prefer nature to take its course. In this case, would the staff be entitled to insist upon responding to the needs of the foetus, even against the mother's wishes? Consider the case of the woman who declines obstetric procedures which are clearly in the best interests of the foetus; for example, the woman who refuses a Caesarian section even though the obstetrician regards this as essential for the baby's welfare.

These are complex issues which have arisen as foetal monitoring devices have become more sensitive, permitting the obstetrician to balance the needs of both mother and foetus in an informed way. To whom is the obstetrician primarily responsible? The question of foetal versus maternal rights is a thorny legal issue at the best of times. In the context of a re-ascendance, in the United States at least, of the anti-abortion lobby, this difficult area may be further clouded by attempts to restrict a woman's right to choose. There can be no substitute for careful understanding of the woman's needs, and reaching a decision on this basis rather than by doctors imposing their own values.

## Postpartum blues

Few women have not heard of or experienced the so-called 'baby blues', characterized by mild depression, anxiety and minimal clouding of consciousness. For most this will be a relatively fleeting experience, although in a minority of cases childbirth may be followed by a more pronounced reaction. The incidence of 'normal' blues has been shown to be anywhere between 50 per cent and 80 per cent (Pitt 1973). The explanation for this is as yet unclear, although because these symptoms are reported to peak around the fourth day, concomitant changes in physiology have been examined. One change that has been shown to coincide is weight loss (Dennis and Blytheway 1965). In a study of daily mood ratings and weight of thirty-seven primiparae, Stein (1980) described synchronous changes in mood and weight. Weight loss has also been described in periodic syndromes of mental disorder, such as the onset of depression, hypomania and catatonia. Although the explanation for weight loss at this time is unclear, since it occurs in the absence of anorexia, it has been linked to increased sodium loss in the urine (Stein *et al.*, 1978), although the cause of the latter is unknown.

Some women can be considered to experience a clinical postnatal depression, as distinct from both the 'baby blues' and the more florid depressive psychoses. Estimates suggest that this problem may affect less than 5 per cent of the population, with the problems persisting in 4 per cent one year after delivery (Pitt 1973). Studies have examined the relationship between depression following the delivery and whether psychological disturbance could be identified antenatally. Women considered clinically depressed following the delivery have been shown to score higher on neuroticism and anxiety scales administered while still pregnant (Meares *et al.* 1976). Elevations in both anxiety and hostility scores were reported by Handley *et al.* (1977). The significance of increased hostility scores is unclear, although they may reflect difficulties in the formation of interpersonal relationships, which may increase vulnerability to depression. It also appeared that 3 of the 7 women severely depressed, and 4 of the 21 mildly depressed, from their sample of 127 women, were depressed antenatally, confirming suggestions by Kumar and Robson (1978), that postnatally depressed women may display depressive symptoms during their pregnancy.

As if depression, albeit transient, were not sufficient, there is evidence to suggest that childbirth is followed by a sharp rise in the incidence of functional psychoses. Kendall *et al.* (1976) studied the influence of childbirth on psychiatric morbidity and found a sharp increase within the first three months after delivery. The rise was largely accounted for by affective psychoses and was too great to have been due to postponement of illnesses that might otherwise have developed during pregnancy. There were also indications of a secondary rise in incidence between nine and twenty-four months following delivery. The reasons for this were unclear, although the authors speculated that the stress associated with mothering, including reduced income and social contacts, may have increased vulnerability at this time, thereby suggesting that the causal mechanisms may be qualitatively different from those responsible for the initial rise.

## The future?

Consideration of postpartum psychoses draws to a close this analysis of the psychological aspects of pregnancy. Having survived, or even flourished, during pregnancy; emerged unscathed, or even sailed through, childbirth; and negotiated the minor and major hurdles of the postpartum period, what next? Some may elect to begin this process again. For others, the disappointments and trials of pregnancy may have deterred them from repetition. The emphasis of the greater part of this book has been on those occasions when something goes wrong; anxiety is high, drugs have been abused, labour is complicated or emotional problems follow the birth. It is natural for such cases to be the object of our clinical attention, since these are the ones which require individual help, but what of the remainder? The assumption of this book has been that for them too, psychological influences may be important and, in the main, are potentially modifiable. They may manifest themselves in subtle ways, in terms of the level of satisfaction with the care received, or more dramatically, as with the baby born displaying foetal alcohol syndrome. In both, psychological processes have exerted an important influence. In the former, staff attention to the psychological needs of the patient may have made the experience a more satisfactory one; the latter is an example of the way in which behavioural aspects of pregnancy may have profound physiological implications. In future greater attention must be brought to bear on such aspects of pregnancy in both medical education and practice. Many benefits may accrue from effective communication between staff and patients (listening and advising), as well as by attempting to engender in the woman a feeling of being actively involved in her care throughout the course of the pregnancy. There may be a tendency to relegate such remarks to the realms of common sense and dismiss them accordingly. Unfortunately, common sense may be seldom common practice. Until such time as prospective studies have documented the impact of attending to psychological factors, such as health behaviour, such considerations may continue to take a subsidiary role compared with the attractions of the technical aspects of care. Time will tell, although the behavioural star appears to be in its ascendancy.

# References

Abel, E. L. (1980) Fetal alcohol syndrome: Behavioural teratology, *Psych. Bull.*, **87**, 29–50.

Adams, M. M., Finley, S. and Hansen, H. et al. (1981) Utilization of prenatal genetic diagnosis in women 35 years of age and older in the US., 1977–1978, *Am. J. Obstet. Gynec.*, **139**, 673–77.

Alberman, E. (1977) Facts and figures, in Chard, T. and Richards, M. (eds), *The Benefits and Hazards of the New Obstetrics*, Lavenham Press, Suffolk.

Artal, R. (1980) Fetal adrenal medulla, *Clin. Obstet. Gynecol.*, **23**, 825–36.

Ascher, B. H. (1978) Maternal anxiety in pregnancy and fetal homeostasis. *JOGN Nurs.*, May/June, 18–21.

Barber, J. (1977) Rapid induction analgesia: A clinical report, *Am. J. Clin. Hypnosis*, **19**, 138–47.

Barber, J. and Adrian-Barber, C. (1982) *Psychological Methods of Pain Control*, Brunner-Mazel, New York.

Baum, D., MacFarlane, A. and Tizard, P. (1977) The benefits and hazards of neonatology, in Chard, T. and Richards, M. (ed), *The Benefits and Hazards of the New Obstetrics*, Lavenham Press, Suffolk.

Beck, N. C. and Hall, D. (1978) Natural childbirth: A review and analysis, *Obstet. Gynecol.*, **52**, 371–9.

Beck, N. C., Siegel, L. J., Davidson, N. P. et al. (1980) The prediction of pregnancy outcome: Maternal preparation, anxiety and attitudinal sets, *J. Psychosom. Res.*, **24**, 343–51.

Becker, M. H. (1974) The health belief model and personal health behaviour, *Hlth. Educ. Monogr.*, **2**, 326–473.

Becker, M. H. (1976) Sociobehavioral determinants of compliance, in Sackett, D. L. and Haynes, R. B. (eds), *Compliance with Therapeutic Regimens*, Johns Hopkins Univ. Press, London.

Beecher, H. K. (1959) *Measurement of Subjective Responses*, Oxford Univ. Press, Oxford.

Bibring, G. L. (1959) Some considerations of the psychological processes in pregnancy, *Psychoanal. Stud. Child.*, **14**, 113–21.

Blackwell, B. (1976) Treatment Adherence, *Brit. J. Psychiat.*, **129**, 513–31.

Bloom, L. J. and Cantrill, D. (1978) Anxiety management training for essential hypertension in pregnancy, *Behav. Ther.*, **9**, 377–82.

Blumberg, B. D., Golbus, M. S. and Hawson, K. H. (1975) The psychological sequelae of abortion performed for a genetic indication, *Am. J. Obstet. Gynec.*, **122**, 799–808.

Bond, M. R. (1971) The relation of pain to the Eysenck Personality Inventory, Cornell Medical Index and Whitely Index of Hypochondriasis. *Br. J. Psychiat.*, **119**, 671–78.

Bond, M. R., Glynn, J. P. and Thomas, D. G. (1976) The relation between pain and personality in patients receiving pentazocine (Fortral) after surgery, *J. Psychosom. Res.*, **20**, 369–81.

Bond, M. R. and Pilowsky, I. (1966) Subjective assessment of pain and its relationship to the administration of analgesics in patients with advanced cancer, *J. Psychosom. Res.*, **10**, 203–6.

Bonica, J. J. (1967) *Principles and Practice of Obstetric Analgesia and Anesthesia*, F. A. Davis, Philadelphia.

Bonica, J. J. (1975) The nature of pain of parturition, *Clin. in Obstet. Gynec.*, **2**, 499–516.

Bonwill, W. G. (1880) Rapid breathing: a pain obtrude in minor surgery, obstetrics. The general practice of medicine and of dentistry, *Philadelphia Medical Times*, p. 10.

Bowker, L. H. (1977) *Drug Use among American Women, Old and Young: Sexual Oppression and Other Drugs*, R and E Research Associates, San Francisco.

Brackbill, Y., Kane, J. and Manniello, R. L. (1974) Obstetric meperidine usage and the assessment of neonatal status, *Anesthesiology*, **40**, 116–20.

Brandes, J. M. (1967) First trimester nausea and vomiting as related to outcome of pregnancy, *Obstet. Gynecol.*, **30**, 427–31.

Breen, D. (1975) *The Birth of a First Child*, Tavistock, London.

Brown, G. W. and Harris, T. (1978) *Social Origins of Depression: A Study of Psychiatric Disorder in Women*, Free Press, New York.

Burns, J. K. (1976) Proceedings: Relationship between blood levels of cortisol and duration of human labour, *J. Physiol.*, **254**, 12pp.

Burstein, I., Kinch, R. A. and Stern, L. (1974) Anxiety, pregnancy, labor and the neonate, *Am. J. Obstet. Gynec.*, **118**, 195–9.

Butler, N. R. and Goldstein, H. (1973) Smoking in pregnancy and subsequent child development, *Br. Med. J.*, **4**, 573–5.

Campbell, S. (1980) Diagnosis of fetal abnormalities by ultrasound, in Milunsky, A. (ed.), *Genetic Disorders and the Fetus*, Plenum Publ. Co., New York.

Campbell, S., Reading, A. E., Cox, D. N. *et al.* (1982) Ultrasound scanning in pregnancy: The short term psychological effects of early real time scans, *J. Psychosom. Obstet. Gynacol.* (in press)

Campbell, S. B. and Taylor, P. M. (1979) Bonding and attachment: Theoretical issues, *Seminars in Perinatology*, **3**, 3–13.

Cartwright, A. (1976) *How Many More Children*, Routledge & Kegan Paul, London.

Cave, C. (1978) Social characteristics of natural childbirth users and nonusers, *Am. J. Pub. Hlth.*, **68**, 898–901.

Chamberlain, R., Chamberlain, G., Howlett, B. and Claireaux, A. (1975), *British Births 1970*, vol. 1, *The First Week of Life*, Heinemann, London.

Chervin, A., Farnsworth, P. B., Freedman, W. L. *et al.* (1977) Amniocentesis for prenatal diagnosis, *N. Y. State*

*J. of Med.*, August, 1406-9.
Clarren, S. K. and Smith, D. W. (1978) The fetal alcohol syndrome, *New Engl. J. Med.*, **298**, 1063-7.
Coffey, T. E. (1966) Ben Street: Gin Lane. Some views of eighteenth-century drinking. *Quart. J. Stud. on Alcohol*, **27**, 669-92.
Cogan, R., Henneburn, W. and Klopfer, F. (1976) Predictors of pain during prepared childbirth, *J. Psychosom. Res.*, **20**, 523-33.
Cohen, F. and Lazurus, R. S. (1973) Active coping dispositions and recovery from surgery, *Psychosom. Med.*, **35**, 375-85.
Cohen, G. (1964) *What's Wrong with Hospitals?*, Penguin Books, London.
Condon, W. S. and Sandler, L. W. (1979) Neonate movement is synchronised with adult speech: Interactional participation and language acquisition, *Science*, **183**, 99-101.
Connolly, A. M., Pancheri, P., Lucchetti, A. *et al.* (1978) in Carenza, L., Pancheri, P. and Zichella, L., (eds), *Clinical Psychoneuroendocrinology in Reproduction*, Academic Press, New York.
Copher, D. E. and Huber, C. P. (1967) Heart rate response of the human fetus to induced maternal hypoxia, *Am. J. Obstet. Gynecol.*, **98**, 320-35.
Coppen, A. J. (1959) Vomiting of early pregnancy, *Lancet*, 24 Jan., 172-3.
Crandon, A. J. (1979) Maternal anxiety and obstetric complications, *J. Psychosom. Res.*, **23**, 109-11.
Cushner, I. M. (1981) Maternal behavior and perinatal risks: Alcohol, smoking and drugs, *Ann. Rev. Publ. Hlth.*, **2**, 201-8.

Dalby, J. T. (1978) Environmental effects on prenatal development, *J. Ped. Psychol.*, **3**, 105-9.
Danaher, B. G., Shisslak, C. M., Thompson, C. B. and Ford, J. O. (1978) A smoking cessation program for pregnant women: An exploratory study, *Am. J. Pub. Hlth.*, **68**, 896-8.
Danziger, S. K. (1979) Treatment of women in childbirth: Implications for family beginnings. *Am. J. Pub. Hlth.*, **9**, 895-901.

Davies, D. P., Gray, O. P., Ellwood, P. C. and Abernethy, M. (1976) Cigarette smoking in pregnancy: Associations with maternal weight gain and foetal growth, *Lancet*, Feb. 385–7.

Dechateau, P. (1979) Effects of hospital practices on synchrony in development of the parent-infant relationship. *Seminars in Perinatology*, **3**, 45–60.

Dennis, K. J. and Blytheway, W. R. (1965) Changes in body weight after delivery, *Br. J. Obstet. Gynaecol.*, **95**, 127.

Deutsch, H. (1943) *The Psychology of Women*, vol. 2, Grune & Stratton, New York.

Dick-Read, G. (1944) *Childbirth Without Fear*, Harper & Bros, New York.

Dick-Read, G. (1972) *Childbirth Without Fear* (rev.), Wessel, H. and Ellis, H. E. (eds), Harper & Row, New York.

Dixson, B., Richards, T. L., Reinsch, S. *et al.* (1981) Midtrimester amniocentesis: Subjective maternal responses, *J. Reproduc. Med.*, **26**, 10–16.

Dobbing, J. (1976) Vulnerable periods in brain growth and somatic growth in Roberts, D. F. (ed.), *The Biology of the Human Foetus*, Taylor & Franusia, London.

Doering, P. L. and Stewart, R. B. (1978) The extent and character of drug consumption during pregnancy, *J. Am. Med. Assoc.*, **239**, 843–6.

Donahue, C. H. and Wan, T. H. (1973) Measuring obstetric risk of prematurity, *Amer. J. Obstet. Gynec.*, **116**, 911–15.

Donovan, J. W. (1977) Randomised controlled trial of anti-smoking advice in pregnancy, *Br. J. Prev. Soc. Med.*, **31**, 6–12.

Dubignon, T., Campbell, D., Curtis, M. and Partington, M. W. (1969) The relation between laboratory measures of sucking, food intake and perinatal factors during the newborn period, *Ch. Devel.*, **40**, 1107–20.

Dunn, H. G., McBurney, A. K., Ingram, S. and Hunter, C. M. (1977) Maternal cigarette smoking during pregnancy and the child's subsequent development: Neurological and intellectual maturation to the age of 6½ years, *Can J. Pub. Hlth.*, **68**, 43–50.


Edwards, K. R. and Jones, M. R. (1970) Personality changes related to pregnancy and obstetric complications,

*Proc. 76th Ann. Conven. Am. Psychol. Assoc.*, 341–3.
Egeland, B. and Vaughn, B. (1981) Failure of bond formation as a cause of abuse, neglect and maltreatment, *Am. J. Orthopsychiat.*, **51**, 78–84.
Eysenck, S. B. G. (1961) Personality and pain assessment in childbirth of married and unmarried mothers, *J. Ment. Sci.*, **107**, 417–30.

Feldstein, M. S. and Butler, N. R. (1965) Analysis of factors affecting perinatal mortality, *Brit. J. Prev. Soc. Med.*, **19**, 128–33.
Ferreira, A. J. (1965) Emotional factors in prenatal environment, *J. Nerv. Ment. Dis.*, **141**, 108–18.
Ferreria, A. J. (1969) *Prenatal Environment*, Charles C. Thomas, Springfield, Illinois.
Fielding, J. E. (1977) Smoking and pregnancy, *New Engl. J. Med.*, **298**, 337–9.
Fielding, J. E. and Yankauer, A. (1978) The pregnant drinker, *New Engl. J. Med.*, **68**, 836–8.
Ford, C. S. (1945) A comparative study of human reproduction, in *Yale University Publications in Anthropology, No. 32*, Yale Univ. Press, New Haven, Conn.
Fordney-Settlage, D. S. (1979) Pelvic examination of women: Genitorectal examination of men, in Green, R. (ed.) *Human Sexuality: A Health Practitioner's Test*, Williams & Wilkins, London.
Forfar, J. O. and Nelson, M. M. (1973) Epidemiology of drug-taking by pregnant women: Drugs that may affect the fetus adversely, *Clin. Pharmac. Theraps.*, **14**, 632–42.
Fox, C. A. (1979) The effects of catecholamines and drug treatment on the fetus and the newborn, *Birth and Fam. J.*, **6**, 157–65.
Fox, C. A. and Knaggs, E. S. (1969) Milk ejection activity (oxytocin) in peripheral venous blood in woman during lactation and in association with coitus, *J. Endocrinol.*, **45**, 145–6.

Goldus, M. S., Longhman, W. D., Epstein, C. J. (1979) Prenatal genetic diagnosis in 3000 amniocentesis, *New Engl. J. Med.*, **300**, 157–61.
Goodlin, R. C. (1973) Sexual activity during pregnancy, *New Engl. J. Med.*, **280**, 379.
Graham, H. (1976) Smoking in pregnancy: The attitudes of

Gynec. Nurs., March/April, 77–80.
Kondas, O. and Scetnicka, B. (1972) Systematic desensitisation as a method of preparation for childbirth, *J. Behav. Ther. Exp. Psychiat.*, **3**, 51–4.
Korner, A. (1971) Individual differences at birth: Implications for early experience and later development. *Am. J. Orthopsychiat.*, **41**, 608–19.
Kosambi, D. D. (1967) Living prehistory in India, *Sci. Amer.*, **216**, 105–15.
Kumar, R. and Robson, K. M. (1978) Previous induced abortion and antenatal depression in primiparae, *Psychol. Med.*, **8**, 711–5.

Lamaze, F. (1958) *Painless Childbirth*, Burke, London.
Langer, E. J., Janis, I. L. and Wolfer, J. A. (1975) Reduction of psychological stress in surgical patients, *J. Exp. Soc. Psychol.*, **11**, 155–65.
Laurence, K. M., James, N., Miller, M. and Campbell, H. (1980) Increased risk of recurrence of pregnancies complicated by foetal neural tube defects in mothers receiving poor diets, and possible benefit of dietary counselling, *Br. Med. J.*, **281**, 1–8.
Lazurus, R. S. (1975) A cognitively oriented psychologist looks at biofeedback, *Am. Psychol.*, **30**, 553–61.
Leboyer, F. (1975) *Birth without Violence*, A. A. Knopf, New York.
Lederman, R. P., Lederman, E., Work, B. A. and McCann, D. C. (1978) The relationship of maternal anxiety, plasma catecholamines and plasma cortisol to progress in labor, *Am. J. Obstet. Gynec.*, **132**, 495–500.
Leifer, A. D., Leiderman, P. H., Barnett, C. and Williams, J. A. (1972) Effects of mother-infant separation on maternal attachment behavior, *Child Devel.*, **43**, 1203–18.
Little, R. E., Grathwohl, H. L., Streissguth, A. P. O., McIntyre, C. (1981) Public awareness and knowledge about the risks of drinking during pregnancy in Multnomah County, Oregon, *Am. J. Pub. Hlth.*, **71**, 312–14.
Little, R. E. and Hook, E. B. (1979) Maternal alcohol and tobacco comsumption and their association with nausea and vomiting during pregnancy, *Acta Obstet. Gynaecol. Scand.*, **58**, 15–17.
Lynch, M. and Roberts, J. (1977) Predicting child abuse:

Signs of bonding failure in the maternity hospital, *Br. Med. J.*, **1**, 624–6.

MacLeod, J. and Gold, R. Z. (1953) The male factor in fertility and sterility. VI semen quality and certain other factors in relation to ease of conception, *Fertil. Steril.*, **4**, 10–33.

Marion, J. P., Kassam, G., Fernhoff, P. M. *et al.* (1980) Acceptance of amniocentesis by low income patients in an urban hospital, *Am. J. Obstet. Gynec.*, **338**, 11–15.

Martin, J. D., Martin, D. C., Lund, C. A. and Streissguth, A. P. (1977) Maternal alcohol ingestion and cigarette smoking and their effects on newborn conditioning, *Alcoholism: Clin. Exp. Res.*, **1** 243–7.

Martin, J. C., Martin, D. C., Sigman, P. and Redon, B. (1978) Offspring survival, development and operant performance following maternal ethanol consumption, *Devel. Psychobiol.*, **10**, 435–46.

Masters, W. H. and Johnson, V. E. (1966) *Human Sexual Response*, Little, Brown, Boston.

McDonald, R. L. (1968) The role of emotional factors in obstetric complications: A review. *Psychosom. Med.*, **30**, 222–43.

McDonald, R. L. and Christakos, A. C. (1963) Relationship of emotional factors during pregnancy to obstetric complications, *Am. J. Obstet. Gynec.*, **86**, 341–8.

McDonald, R. L. and Parham, K. J. (1964) Relation of emotional changes during pregnancy to obstetric complications in unmarried primigravidae, *Am. J. Obstet. Gynec.*, **90**, 195–9.

McFarlane, A. (1974) If a smile is so important, *New Scientist*, **62**, 164–6.

McKinlay, J. B. (1970) The new latecomers for antenatal care, *Br. J. Prev. Soc. Med.*, **24**, 52–7.

Mead, M. and Newton, N. (1967) Cultural patterning of perinatal behavior, in Richardson, S. A. and Guttmacher, A. F. (eds), *Childbearing: Its Social and Psychological Aspects*, Williams & Wilkins, Baltimore.

Meares, R., Grinwade, J. and Wood, C. (1976) A possible relationship between anxiety in pregnancy and puerperal depression, *J. Psychosom. Res.*, **20**, 605–10.

Melzack, R. (1973) *The Puzzle of Pain*, Penguin, London.

Melzack, R., Weisz, A. Z. and Sprague, T. L. (1963). Strategems for controlling pain: Contributions of auditory stimulation and suggestion, *Exper. Neurol.*, **8**, 239.

Meyer, M. B. (1978) How does maternal smoking affect birth weight and maternal weight gain?, *Am. J. Obstet. Gynecol.*, **131**, 888–93.

Milne, L. S. and Rich, O. J. (1981) Cognitive and affective aspects of the responses of pregnant women to sonography, *Mat. Ch. Nurs. J.*, March/April, 15–39.

Morishima, H. O., Pederson, H. and Finser, M. (1978) The influence of maternal psychological stress on the fetus, *Am. J. Obstet. Gynec.*, **131**, 286–90.

Nelson, N. M., Enkin, M. W., Saigal, S. *et al.*, (1980) A randomized clinical trial of the Leboyer approach to childbirth, *New Engl. J. Med.*, **302**, 655–60.

Netterbladt, P., Fagerstrum, C. F. and Uddenberg, N. (1976) The significance of reported childbirth pain, *J. Psychosom. Res.*, **20**, 215–21.

Neutra, R. R., Fienberg, S. E., Greenland, S. and Friedman, E. A. (1978) Effect of fetal monitoring on neonatal death rates, *New Engl. J. Med.*, **299**, 324–6.

Newton, N. and Newton, M. (1962) Mothers' reactions to their newborn babies, *J. Am. Med. Assoc.*, **181**, 206–13.

Newton, R. W., Webster, P. A., Maskrey, N. and Phillips, A. B. (1979) Psychosocial stress in pregnancy and its relation to the onset on premature labour, *Br. Med. J.*, August, 411–13.

Norr, K. L. Block, C. R., Charles, A. *et al.* (1977) Explaining pain and enjoyment in childbirth, *J. Hlth. Soc. Behav.*, **18**, 260–75.

Nuckolls, K. B., Cassel, J. and Kaplan, B. H. (1972) Psychosocial assets, life crisis and the prognosis of pregnancy. *Am. J. Epidemiol.*, **95**, 431–41.

Oakley, A. (1977) Cross-cultural practices, in Chard, T. and Richards, M. (eds), *The Benefits and Hazards of the New Obstetrics*, Lavenham Press, Suffolk.

O'Connor, S. M., Vietze, P. M. and Hopkins, J. B. (1977) Postpartum extended maternal infant contact: Subsequent mothering and childcare. Presented at the Society for Pediatric Research, San Francisco (unpublished).

Pancheri, P., Ermini, M., Fiore, V. et al. (1979) Psychoneuroendocrine correlates in labour, in Zichella, L. and Pancheri, P. (eds), *Psychoneuroendocrine in Reproduction*, Elsevier, Holland, pp. 575–88.

Parke, R., Power, T. G., Tinsley, B. R. and Hymel, S. (1979) The father's role in the family system. *Sems in Perinat.*, **3**, 25–34.

Peppers, L. G. and Knapp, R. J. (1980) Maternal reactions to involuntary fetal/infant death, *Psychiatry*, **43**, 155–9.

Persson, P. H., Grennert, L., Gennser, G., and Kullander. S. (1976) A study of smoking and pregnancy with special reference to foetal growth, *Acta Obstet. Gynaecol. Scand., Suppl.*, **78**, 33–9.

Pitt, B. (1973) Maternity blues, *Br. J. Psychiat.*, **122**, 431–3.

Quick, J. D., Greenlick, M. R. and Roghmann, K. J. (1981) Prenatal care and pregnancy outcomes in an HMO and general population: A multivariate cohort analysis, *Am. J. Pub. Hlth.*, **71**, 381–90.

Rachman, S. (1974) *The Meaning of Fear*, Penguin, London.

Reading, A. E. (1983) Bonding: An evaluation of the concept and its implications for obstetric practice, in Studd, J. W. (ed.), *Progress in Obstetrics and Gynaecology*, vol. 3, Churchill Livingstone, Edinburgh.

Reading, A. E. (1982) The management of fear related to vaginal examination, *J. Psychosom. Obstet. Gynaecol.*, (in press).

Reading, A. E. (1979) The short-term effects of psychological preparation for surgery, *Soc. Sci. Med.*, **13A**, 641–54.

Reading, A. E., Campbell, S., Cox, D. N. and Sledmere, C. M. (1982a) Health beliefs and health care behaviors in pregnancy, *Psychol. Med.*, **12**, 379–83.

Reading, A. E., Sledmere, C. M., Cox, D. N. and Campbell, S. (1982b) How women view their post-episiotomy pain, *Br. Med. J.*, **284**, 243–6.

Reid, M. E. and McIlwaine, G. M. (1980) Consumer opinion of a hospital antenatal clinic, *Soc. Sci. Med.*, **14A**, 363–8.

Robson, K. M. and Kumar, R. (1980) Delayed onset of maternal affection after childbirth, *Br. J. Psychiat.*, **136**,

347–53.

Rodeck, C. H. and Campbell, S. (1979). The early prenatal diagnosis of neural tube defects. *Trends in Neurosci.*, Nov., 1–4.

Rosen, M. (1977) Pain and its relief, in Chard, T. and Richards, M. (eds), *The Benefits and Hazards of the New Obstetrics*, Lavenham Press, Suffolk.

Rutter, M. (1979) Separation experiences: A new look at an old topic, *J. Pediat.*, **95**, 147–54.

Rybstein-Blinchik, E. (1979) Effects of different cognitive strategies on chronic pain experience, *J. Behav. Med.*, **2**, 93–101.

Sahu, S. (1981) Coping with perinatal death, *J. Reprod. Med.*, **26**, 129–32.

Scanlon, J. W. (1976) Effects of local anesthetics administered to parturient women on the neurological and behavioral performance of newborn children, *Bull. N.Y. Acad. Med.*, **52**, 231–40.

Shereshefsky, P. M. and Yarrow, L. J. (eds) (1973) *Psychological Aspects of a First Pregnancy and Early Postnatal Adaptation*, Raven Press, New York.

Sime, A. M. (1976) Relationships of preoperative fear, type of coping and information received about surgery, *J. Consult. Clin. Psychol.*, **44**, 716–24.

Smithells, R., Sheppard, S. and Achorah, C. (1976) Vitamin deficiencies and neural tube defects, *Arch. Dis. Child.*, **51**, 944–50.

Solberg, D. A., Butler, J. and Wagner, N. N. (1973) Sexual behavior in pregnancy, *New Engl. J. Med.*, **288**, 1098–1103.

Spielberger, C. D., Gorsuch, R. L. and Lushene, R. E. (1970) *The State Trait Anxiety Inventory*, Consulting Psychologists Press, Palo Alto, Ca.

Spielberger, C. D., and Jacobs, G. A. (1979) Emotional reactions to the stress of pregnancy and obstetric complications, in Carenza, L. and Zichella, L. (eds), *Emotion and Reproduction*, Academic Press, London, pp. 13–24.

Stachnik, T. J. (1980) Priorities for psychology in medical education and health care delivery, *Am. Psychol.*, **35**, 8–15.

Starkman, M. N. (1976) Psychological responses to the use of the fetal monitor during labor, *Psychosom. Med.*, **38**, 269–77.

Stein, G. S. (1980) The pattern of mental change and body weight change in the first postpartum week. *J. Psychosom. Res.*, **24**, 165–71.

Stein, G. S., Milton, F., Bebbington, P. *et al.* (1978) The relationship between mood disturbance and free and total plasma tryptophan in postpartum women, *Br. Med. J.*, **2**, 637–9.

Stein, Z., Susser, M., Warburton, D. *et al.* (1975) Spontaneous abortion as a screening device: The effect of fetal survival on the incidence of birth defects, *Am. J. Epidemiol.*, **102**, 275–90.

Stimson, G. V. (1974) Obeying doctor's orders: A view from the other side. *Soc. Sci. Med.*, **8**, 97–104.

Tolor, A. and DiGrazia, P. V. (1976) Sexual attitudes and behavior patterns during and following pregnancy, *Arch. Sex Behav.*, **5**, 539–51.

Towers, B. (1981) Medical experiments on human beings, *J. Med. Ethics*, **7**, 19–23.

Turnbull, A. C. (1977) Introduction, in Chard, T. and Richards, M. (eds), *The Benefits and Hazards of the New Obstetrics*, Lavenham Press, Suffolk.

Uddenberg, N., Nilsson, A. and Almeren, P. I. (1971) Navsea in pregnancy: psychological and psychosomatic aspects, *J. Psychosom. Res.*, **15**, 269–75.

Uddenberg. N., Fagerstrom, C. F. and Zannders, M. H. (1976) Reproductive conflicts, mental symptoms and time labour, *J. Psychosom. Res.* **20**, 575–81.

Ungerleider, J. T., Andrysiak, T., Fairbanks, L. *et al.* (1981) Cancer chemotherapy and marijuana, *UCLA Cancer Center Bull.*, **8**, 3–6.

Vermeesch, J. (1977) Maternal nutrition and outcome of pregnancy, in Worthington, B. S., Vermeesch, J. and Williams, S. R. (eds), *Nutrition in Pregnancy and Lactation*. C. V. Mosby, St. Louis.

Vevovsky, I., Platonov. K., Plotcher, V. and Shugom, E. (eds) (1960) *Painless Childbirth through Psychoprophy-*

*laxis*, Moscow Foreign Languages Publishing House, Moscow.

Vincent, P. (1961) *Recherches sur la fecondité biologique*, Presses Universitaires de France, Paris.

Wagner, N. N., Butler, J. C. and Sanders, J. P. (1976) Prematurity and orgasmic coitus during pregnancy. Data on a small sample, *Fertil. Steril.*, **27**, 911–15.

Waletzky, L. R. (1979) Husbands' problems with breastfeeding, *Am. J. Orthopsychiat.*, **49**, 349–52.

Weinstein, L. (1980) Breast milk – A natural resource, *Am. J. Obstet. Gynec.*, **136**, 973–5.

Werts, C. E., Gardiner, S. H., Mitchell, K. *et al.* (1965) Factors related to behavior in labor, *J. Hlth. Human Behav.*, **6**, 238–42.

Williamson, E. M. (1965) Incidence and family aggregation of major congenital malformations of the central nervous system, *J. Med. Genet.*, **2**, 161–72.

Williams, C. C., Williams, R. A., Griswold, M. J. and Holmes, T. H. (1975) Pregnancy and life change, *J. Psychosom. Res.*, **19**, 123–9.

Wilson, M. E., Gilman, J. A. and Kellogg, B. (1979) Prenatal diagnosis by amniocentesis in 800 pregnancies, *West. J. Med.*, **131**, 201–4.

Wilson, R. W. and Schifrin, B. S. (1980) Is any pregnancy low risk? *Obstet. Gynec.*, **55**, 653–6.

Winnicott, D. W. (1958) *Collected Papers*, Basic Books, New York.

Wolkind, S. and Zajicek, E. (1981) *Pregnancy: A Psychological and Social Study*, Academic Press, London.

Worthington, B. S. (1979) Nutrition in pregnancy: Some current concepts and questions, *Birth and Family J.*, **6**, 181–92.

# Index

abortion, 3, 23, 33, 34, 35, 57–8, 60, 68, 107
alcohol, 22, 25–6, 29, 32–5, 39, 40–1, 47, 48, 50, 104
amniocentesis, 53–4, 56–60
antenatal clinic attendance, 27–9, 60
antenatal foetal diagnosis, 28, 53–69, 106–7
antiemetics, 47
anxiety
  effects of, 10–24
  management, 23
  over pregnancy, 49, 76
  over vaginal examination, 3, 29
attachment, *see* bonding

bonding
  mother–foetus, 60
  mother–infant, 8, 43, 47, 82, 88–102
breast feeding, 92–4, 97–9, 100

child abuse, 91
childlessness, 6
compliance, 9, 22, 25–6, 50, 104, 109–10
contraception, 2–3, 76, 97
couvade, 75

death of foetus/neonate, 99–100
delivery, 7–8, 10, 11–15, 68, 70–1, 74–87, 89–96, 101–2, 104–5
depression, 1, 107–9
diet, 22, 25, 30, 35–7
drugs
  abuse of, 37–8

epidural anaesthesia, 79, 82, 83
episiotomy, 83, 96, 104–6
extended contact between mother and neonate, 91–4

father *see* partner
fecundability, 3–4
foetal alcohol syndrome, 25, 32, 34, 35
foetal monitors, 7, 66–7, 69
foetal movement perception, 40, 47–9, 58
foetoscopy, 53, 54

genetic counselling, 58

health advice, 22, 25, 35, 40, 50, 104, 109–10
health beliefs, 39–40
husband *see* partner
hypnosis, 85

# Index

infertility, 4–5

labour
  cultural influences, 7–8, 74–5, 96
  difficulties, 12–13, 20–1, 81
  prematurity, 15, 21, 83, 94

Manifest Anxiety Scale, 12, 13
marriage (effects of pregnancy), 44
miscarriage *see* death

nausea, 45–7
neonatal behaviour, 92–4
neonatal health, 30–7, 82–3
neonate, mother's reaction, 94–6
neural tube defects, 36–7
nutrition *see* diet

pain
  anxiety, 76–7, 78
  attitudes, 76
  labour, 69, 70–1, 74–6
  meaning, 73–4
  mechanisms, 80–1
  medication, 79–80, 81–3, 86–7, 95
  personality, 77–8
  psychological control, 83–6
  understanding, 72–3
partner role of, 46, 61, 69, 85, 98–9, 100, 101–2, 104
postpartum blues *see* depression
postpartum psychosis, 8, 108

prematurity, 15, 21
preparation for birth, 84–6
psychosocial support, 14, 19

quickening *see* foetal movement perception

relaxation, 85

separation of mother–baby, 90–2, 101
sexual behaviour, 3–4, 5, 50–2, 105–6
smoking, 22, 25–6, 29–32, 33, 34, 39, 40–1, 47, 48, 50, 104
State–Trait Anxiety Inventory, 12, 13
still birth *see* death
stress, 5, 11, 19, 22, 95, 96, 103
stress hormones, 20–1, 22
stressful life events, 14–15, 23

technology and psychological impact, 6–8, 55–6, 67–9, 106
teenage pregnancy, 2–3, 28
termination of pregnancy *see* abortion
trait anxiety, 5, 12, 16, 19

ultrasound feedback and psychological effects, 40, 49–50, 60–6
ultrasound examination, 48–9, 53, 54–5, 68–9